THE EVERYTHING®
HEALTH GUIDE TO
Migraines

Dear Reader,

Migraines hurt. Not just physically, but emotionally, socially, and even financially. Left untreated or improperly treated, this debilitating neurological condition diminishes overall quality of life. Fortunately, there are many treatment options available to stop migraine pain and even prevent migraine attacks. But a huge proportion of migraineurs remain undiagnosed or untreated simply because they don't have the knowledge they need to seek help.

As a person who has dealt with debilitating migraines since childhood, I know just how frustrating misperceptions of a migraine as "just a headache" can be. Even getting an accurate diagnosis can be a challenge; the public perception of head pain can cause us to downplay the condition for many years, and not all physicians have sufficient skills and experience in headache medicine.

And as a medical writer and editor and a patient advocate, I have discovered that empowering people with timely, accurate, and easy-to-understand information about their health is the best way to motivate them toward better care. An informed patient knows what questions to ask, works with her doctor to set and achieve treatment goals, and doesn't settle for less when it comes to her health.

Remember—you alone have the power and the responsibility, to manage your own health. I hope you will find this book a useful reference in getting the diagnosis and care you deserve.

Sincerely,

Paula Ford-Martin

THE

EVERYTHING
Series

THE EVERYTHING® HEALTH GUIDES are a part of the bestselling Every-thing® series and cover important health topics like anxiety, postpartum care, and thyroid disease. Packed with the most recent, up-to-date data, THE EVERYTHING® HEALTH GUIDES help you get the right diagnosis, choose the best doctor, and find the treatment options that work for you. With this one comprehensive resource, you and your family members have all the information you need right at your fingertips.

 Alerts: Urgent warnings

 Essentials: Quick, handy tips

 Facts: Important snippets of information

 Questions: Answers to common problems

When you're done reading, you can finally
say you know **EVERYTHING®**!

DIRECTOR OF INNOVATION Paula Munier

EXECUTIVE EDITOR, SERIES BOOKS Brielle K. Matson

MANAGING EDITOR, EVERYTHING SERIES Lisa Laing

COPY CHIEF Casey Ebert

ACQUISITIONS EDITOR Katie McDonough

DEVELOPMENT EDITOR Brett Palana-Shanahan

Visit the entire Everything® series at *www.everything.com*

THE
EVERYTHING®

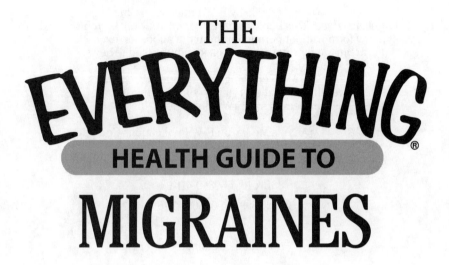

HEALTH GUIDE TO

MIGRAINES

Professional advice to help ease the pain
and find the solution that's right for you

Paula Ford-Martin

Technical Review by Daniel H. Lachance, M.D.

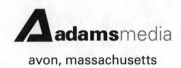

avon, massachusetts

st girls—Kate and Cassie

• • •

An Everything® Series Book.
Everything® and everything.com® are registered
trademarks of F+W Publications, Inc.

Published by Adams Media, an F+W Publications Company
57 Littlefield Street, Avon, MA 02322 U.S.A.
www.adamsmedia.com

ISBN 10: 1-59869-411-1

ISBN 13: 978-1-59869-411-6

Printed in Canada.

J I H G F E D C B A

Library of Congress Cataloging-in-Publication Data
is available from the publisher.

This publication is designed to provide accurate and authoritative information
with regard to the subject matter covered. It is sold with the understanding that
the publisher is not engaged in rendering legal, accounting, or other professional advice. If legal advice or other expert assistance is required, the services
of a competent professional person should be sought.
—From a *Declaration of Principles* jointly adopted by a Committee of the
American Bar Association and a Committee of Publishers and Associations

Many of the designations used by manufacturers and sellers to distinguish their
products are claimed as trademarks. Where those designations appear in this
book and Adams Media was aware of a trademark claim, the designations have
been printed with initial capital letters.

The Everything® Health Guide to Migraines is intended as a reference volume
only, not as a medical manual. In light of the complex, individual, and specific nature of health problems, this book is not intended to replace professional medical advice. The ideas, procedures, and suggestions in this book are
intended to supplement, not replace, the advice of a trained medical professional. Consult your physician before adopting the suggestions in this book, as
well as about any condition that may require diagnosis or medical attention.
The author and publisher disclaim any liability arising directly or indirectly
from the use of this book.

This book is available at quantity discounts for bulk purchases.
For information, please call 1-800-289-0963.

*All the examples and dialogues used in this book are fictional and have
been created by the author to illustrate medical situations.*

Contents

Acknowledgments

An enormous debt of gratitude is owed to Shana Priwer and Cynthia Phillips, both top-notch writers and researchers who contributed considerable expertise, time, and knowledge to this book and spent many late nights making it a reality. It was a privilege to work with you. I'd also like to acknowledge Dr. Daniel Lachance for lending his clinical expertise to this project. Thanks go to my two beautiful daughters—Cassie and Kate—for their patience, love, and support throughout the process. And speaking of patience, I'd like to extend my appreciation to Katie McDonough, Brielle Matson, and everyone at Adams Media for your understanding and guidance. Finally, a shout out to my agent Barb Doyen, master negotiator and head cheerleader, without whom this book would not be possible.

Introduction

WHETHER YOU'VE BEEN diagnosed with chronic migraines, think you may have the condition, or care about someone who does, you'll find *The Everything® Health Guide to Migraines* an important guidebook to improving physical and emotional well-being. The impact of migraine goes well beyond the attack period; it can have far-reaching repercussions at work and home, and it can affect every facet of your life, from the food you eat to the social activities you choose to participate in.

Migraine is a painful and debilitating neurological condition that costs Americans billions of dollars in health care spending, lost workplace productivity, and reduced quality of life. More than "just a headache," a migraine attack is a severe episode of prolonged head pain that is frequently accompanied by nausea, vomiting, visual disturbances, sensitivity to light and sound, sensory changes, and mental confusion. And migraine doesn't begin, or end, with head pain. A migraine attack is often preceded and/or followed by a constellation of symptoms, and the entire episode may span a period of several debilitating days. This can result in significant disability for anyone experiencing frequent migraine episodes.

Migraineurs—those people living with chronic migraines— come in all shapes and sizes. While women are three times as likely to experience migraine as men, the condition can strike men and women, young and old. It's estimated that 28 million Americans have experienced a migraine headache. And more than half remain undiagnosed—either due to a misdiagnosis or a reluctance to seek help. Getting a proper diagnosis may well be the most challenging step of migraine care.

There is a wide spectrum of effective treatments available for migraine, from acute analgesics that treat an attack already in progress to prophylactic medications that prevent migraines from occurring in the first place. Some complementary therapies, including acupuncture and certain vitamins and herbal supplements, have also shown promise, as have biofeedback and progressive relaxation. And there are exciting and promising new therapies on the research horizon.

Knowledge is your most important tool in managing this condition. Documenting your migraines with a headache diary, identifying potential triggers that may be causing your attacks, staying abreast of new treatment and research developments, understanding your treatment regimen, and being a smart health care consumer all contribute to successful outcomes for the migraineur. Knowing how to find an experienced health care provider who will be a partner in your care is also key. This book contains all these tools, along with practical information on lifestyle and advocacy issues surrounding migraine disease.

Living with a chronic condition can be emotionally difficult for both you and your friends and family. Migraineurs may experience depression or anxiety as a result of their condition, and healthy coping may become a challenge. This is why it's important to have a support network; again, knowledge makes things just a little easier. Share this book with those people that you care for so they can understand both the health and lifestyle implications of migraine and get tips on how they can help you survive, and even thrive, with chronic migraine.

CHAPTER 1

Migraine Basics

EVERY DAY, WORLDWIDE, over 19 million migraine attacks occur— 900,000 in the United States alone. Migraines are painful headache episodes, sometimes accompanied by visual and other sensory disturbances, which are caused by chemical, electrical, and vascular changes in the brain. They can last up to three days and frequently incapacitate the migraineur, or migraine sufferer. Despite the availability of new and effective preventative drugs and painkillers, migraine continues to be one of the most underdiagnosed and undertreated conditions in America.

Migraine by the Numbers

An estimated 28 million Americans, or 12 percent of the U.S. population, suffer from migraines. Adult women are roughly three times more likely to suffer from migraine than men; one in five women experience migraine headaches versus one in twenty men. The condition occurs most commonly between the ages of fifteen to fifty-five, and migraine occurrence seems to diminish with age; adults age eighteen to forty-four were nearly three times as likely to report suffering a migraine or severe headache over the past three months than adults age sixty-five or older.

Migraine is also an expensive disease. A 2006 survey found that migraines cost American health care and business a staggering $24 billion each year. This includes direct medical expenditures for migraine care (i.e., prescription drugs, emergency room care, and inpatient and outpatient treatment) of over $12 billion. In addition, American employers lose another $12 billion each year from employee absences, short-term disability insurance, and workers' compensation claims—and that doesn't include costs for lost productivity of employees who go to work during a migraine episode.

That cost may be exacerbated by the fact that many people living with migraine do not have adequate prescription drug insurance coverage. In a study of patients who used prescription triptan medication for migraine relief, 42 percent of those surveyed said that their insurance did not cover enough monthly medication to treat their migraine, and 37 percent had not filled a triptan prescription because of the out-of-pocket cost.

 Fact

During a migraine attack, men and women spend 4.5 hours and 6 hours confined to bed, respectively. Over the course of a year, that translates to about 3.8 bedridden days for men and 5.6 bedridden days for women, and over 112 million bedridden days for the total American migraine population.

Underdiagnosed

The American Migraine Prevalence and Prevention Study (AMPP), a large-scale, population-based epidemiological study of migraine and migraine prevention commissioned by the National Headache Foundation, found that only an estimated 48 percent of people with migraine symptoms receive the correct diagnosis. Among women, the percentage may be even lower.

The stereotypes and stigmas associated with migraine may prevent women from seeking help. Historically, headache pain has often been discounted as a legitimate medical condition. Patients may dismiss migraine symptoms as "just a headache" and fail to seek help. The fact that migraine often coexists with mood disorders like depression and anxiety may also contribute to this problem.

Migraineurs may hesitate to seek help because of the fear that they'll be considered psychologically unstable or not taken seriously. Research shows, however, that migraine is clearly not a psychiatric or psychological condition—it is a biological brain disorder.

Some of the fault for the high underdiagnosis rate of migraine lies with the health care provider. Primary care physicians may not be knowledgeable in the diagnosis and treatment of the condition or familiar with the criteria. According to one study, less than half of internal medicine residents and 62 percent of family practice residents consider themselves prepared to treat patients with headache.

Many undiagnosed migraineurs are actually *misdiagnosed* with other types of headache. One study found that sinus headache was the clinical diagnosis given in 42 percent of migraine cases, and tension headache was the diagnosis in 32 percent of migraine cases. A patient's assertion that they believe they have sinus or tension headaches seemed to be a strong factor in misdiagnosis by doctors.

Undertreated

Migraine also seems to be undertreated, with more than half of migraine sufferers relying on over-the-counter pain relievers or simply toughing it out with no drugs at all to treat their migraine headache. Over 40 percent have never used preventative therapies such as propranolol (Inderal), topiramate (Topamax), and divalproex sodium (Depakote) to treat a migraine attack, although these drugs have been proven to significantly decrease migraine occurrence, severity, and duration. And an estimated 60 percent use over-the-counter treatments only to ease the pain of migraine. Overuse of some OTC treatments can result in rebound headaches, resulting in a constant cycle of headache pain (for more on rebound headaches, see page 98).

With such effective treatments available to ease this debilitating condition, why do so many people continue to suffer the pain and poor quality of life associated with migraine? Sometimes, migraineurs who have had a bad previous experience with a doctor or course of drugs will attempt to self-treat the condition. The patient may discontinue a medication due to side effects, unaware that dosage adjustments or other medications are an option. Or, the patient and doctor may not be up-to-date on the available therapies. Understanding the nature of your condition and the choices available to you are key to getting the best possible care.

 Fact

A 2006 study of adult migraineurs published in the journal *Head-ache* found that African American patients studied were less likely to receive a migraine diagnosis and/or treatment than their Caucasian counterparts. They were also less likely to seek out professional care for head pain and reported lower levels of trust in doctors.

Types of Migraine

Migraine is classified by two major types—migraine with aura and migraine without aura. An aura is a group of changes that proceed a migraine headache, including visual, sensory, and cognitive changes. Both types share some common features, including a duration of roughly four to seventy-two hours and a one-sided, pulsating headache that worsens with even light physical activity.

Around 80 percent of migraineurs have migraine without aura, also called common migraine. Their headache begins without the "early warning system" of the aura. However, some people with this type of migraine may experience a prodrome—a group of physical and/or emotional symptoms occurring up to seventy-two hours before a migraine headache (see page 8 for more on prodromes).

The International Headache Society (IHS), a worldwide organization for clinicians involved with the study of headache, has established diagnostic guidelines for migraine that have been adapted by most health care practice organizations worldwide, including the American Academy of Neurology.

The IHS criteria for a diagnosis of migraine without aura is at least five attacks fulfilling the following:

- Headache attacks lasting four to seventy-two hours (untreated or unsuccessfully treated)
- Headache has at least two of the following characteristics:
  - Primarily felt on one side of the head (although referred pain may be felt anywhere on the face or head)
  - Pulsating or throbbing quality
  - Moderate to severe pain intensity
  - Aggravation by or causing avoidance of routine physical activity (e.g., walking or climbing stairs)
- During headache at least one of the following occurs:
  - Nausea and/or vomiting
  - Sensitivity to light and sound (photophobia and phonophobia)
- Headache is not attributed to another neurological or physical disorder

Those patients who meet all the above criteria but have experienced fewer than five attacks are usually diagnosed with "probable migraine without aura." Migraine attacks that occur for fifteen or more days of the month for at least three consecutive months are considered to be "chronic migraine without aura."

Migraine with Aura

Migraine with aura is sometimes referred to as a *classic migraine*. The most common type of aura is visual. Migraine with aura is experienced by roughly 20 percent of all migraineurs.

The IHS criteria for a diagnosis of migraine with aura is at least two attacks fulfilling the following criteria:

- Aura consisting of at least one of the following fully reversible symptoms, but no motor weakness:

- Visual symptoms including positive features (e.g., flickering lights, spots, or lines) and/or negative features (i.e., loss of vision)
- Sensory symptoms including positive features (i.e., pins and needles) and/or negative features (i.e., numbness)
- Dysphasic speech disturbance (difficulty speaking)
- At least two of the following:
  - Homonomous (affecting one-half of the visual fields of both eyes) visual symptoms and/or unilateral (or one sided) sensory symptoms (e.g., tingling of the arm)
  - At least one aura symptom develops gradually over five minutes and/or different aura symptoms occur in succession over five minutes
  - Each symptom lasts more than five and less than sixty minutes
- Headache attacks lasting four to seventy-two hours (untreated or unsuccessfully treated)
- Headache begins during the aura or follows aura within sixty minutes and has at least two of the following characteristics:
  - Primarily felt on one side of the head (although referred pain may be felt anywhere on the face or head)
  - Pulsating or throbbing quality
  - Moderate to severe pain intensity
  - Aggravation by or causing avoidance of routine physical activity (e.g., walking or climbing stairs)
- During headache at least one of the following occurs:
  - Nausea and/or vomiting
  - Sensitivity to light and sound (photophobia and phonophobia)
- Headache is not attributed to another disorder

There are some uncommon health conditions that may mimic migraine with aura. For this reason, your physician will take a complete health history and perform a physical and neurological exam to rule out other causes of aura and headache. The diagnostic process is described in detail in Chapter 3.

Less Common Types of Migraine

Finally, there are several less common classes of migraine that fall outside of the two major classes described previously. These are:

- **Basilar Migraine:** A migraine with aura causing neurological dysfunction in the area of the brain supplied by the basilar artery, the brainstem. It has a specific aura profile, and the migraine pain affects both sides of the head.
- **Familial Hemiplegic Migraine:** A severe but rare migraine with aura that causes weakness or paralysis on one side of the body and can result in coma.
- **Retinal (or Ocular) Migraine:** A rare type of migraine associated with blindness or blurred vision in one eye for an extended period (to be distinguished from typical migraine aura which upon careful assessment involves the same points in the visual field of both eyes for five to thirty minutes).
- **Abdominal Migraine:** Most common in children, abdominal migraine is characterized by bouts of abdominal pain, nausea, and vomiting that can last for up to seventy-two hours.
- **Migraine Aura Without Headache:** In this type of migraine, the typical visual and neurological symptoms of aura occur, but there is no headache that follows.

Anatomy of a Migraine

A migraine progresses through four distinct phases: prodrome, aura, headache, and postheadache (or postdrome). Not every migraineur will experience every phase; some don't have auras and others don't have a prodrome. The feature virtually all share is the headache phase, which can last anywhere from four hours to three days. Rarely, some people experience a migraine aura without headache.

Prodrome

Symptoms that anticipate the start of a migraine attack are known as the prodrome phase of the migraine. Not everyone experiences a prodrome—it's estimated that between 25 and 60 percent of migraineurs experience prodromal symptoms anywhere from one to twenty-four hours prior to a migraine attack. Prodrome can occur in both migraine with aura and migraine without aura.

Prodromal symptoms can be physical and mental in nature. The most common reported symptoms are fatigue and mood changes such as irritability, depression, and euphoria. Gastrointestinal symptoms such as diarrhea, constipation, and stomach pain are also reported. Other prodromal symptoms include neck pain, sensitivity to smell and light, hearing loss, dizziness, yawning, weakness, food cravings, tingling of the head and/or extremities, and nose and sinus problems. Migraineurs may experience some, all, or none of these symptoms.

Essential

Triptan drugs such as sumatriptan (Imitrex), zolmitriptan (Zomig), and eletriptan (Relpax) may be useful in preventing a migraine headache if taken during the prodromal phase. For people with a short prodromal phase (two hours or less), a rapid-acting triptan like rizatriptan (Maxalt) may be recommended.

Aura

An estimated 20 percent of people with migraine experience an aura before or during headache. Aura symptoms can vary dramatically from person to person and can include tingling and/or numbness in the fingers, difficulty speaking or coming up with the right word (known as *dysphasia*), and motor weakness. The most common type of aura is visual disturbance. This often occurs as flickering spots or lines or areas of loss of vision. Imaging studies have shown that during a migraine aura, changes occur in blood flow to the brain and cerebral metabolic activity (see All about Auras section, page 12).

Headache

Migraine headache pain is triggered by a complex cascade of neurochemical and inflammatory responses involving the brainstem and vascular structures in the head. The pain usually occurs on one side of the head, often around the eye or temple, and is typically described as throbbing or pulsating. Migraine pain builds in intensity as the headache progresses and may generalize to involve both sides of the head. Physical activity—even routine movement such as standing from a sitting position, climbing stairs, or bending over to pick something up—intensifies the discomfort.

During the headache phase of migraine, the migraineur may experience heightened sensitivity to light and sound. Stomach upset is also very common; for this reason medications that stop nausea and vomiting (antiemetics) are frequently prescribed to migraineurs. Migraine headaches—both with and without aura—can last anywhere from four hours to three days, sometimes persisting through sleep.

Postdrome

Once the head pain of migraine resolves, patients may experience what is known as the *postdrome*—or what some migraineurs call the headache hangover. This phase may last anywhere from a few hours to more than a day. Fatigue, cognitive difficulties, mood change, dizziness, weakness, and a low-grade headache are all common features of postdrome. Because all of these symptoms may initially appear during migraine headache or even before the headache during prodrome, researchers aren't sure whether postdrome is a distinct phenomenon or if it's just a continuation and lessening of headache symptoms.

There have been only a few clinical studies of postdromes, but they seem to indicate that patients who experience a postdrome tend to have higher intensity migraine pain and more migraine triggers. They also are more likely to experience prodrome and aura.

What Is Known, and Not Known

What makes one person more likely to develop migraine than another is not completely and clearly understood. While having a family history of migraine greatly increases the odds of developing the condition, certain environmental factors such as socioeconomic status and stress have also been linked to migraine disease. It's likely that a combination of both genetic predisposition and environmental triggers cause migraine.

Some risk factors that are associated with an increased risk of migraine include:

- **Heredity**. Between 70 and 80 percent of people with migraine have a family history of the condition.
- **Gender and age**. After puberty, migraine is two to three times more common in women and peaks in the thirties and forties.
- **Race**. Caucasians are more likely to develop migraine than African Americans or people of Asian descent.

 Alert

Migraine also increases your risk of developing a number of physical and psychological disorders, including epilepsy, certain sleep disorders, asthma, Raynaud's disease, depression, and panic disorder. See Chapter 19 for more information on these comorbidities.

Genetics and Heredity

Family history does play a role in migraine. Studies of families and twins have shown that migraine risk is much higher when there is a first-degree relative with a history of migraine, even when family members lived apart. This connection is particularly strong in the case of migraine with aura.

According to the National Headache Foundation, four out of five migraineurs report a family history of migraine. A child who has one parent with migraine has a 50 percent chance of developing the condition; if both parents have migraine the chance of the child developing migraine raises to 75 percent.

Researchers have not yet isolated the genes associated with migraine with aura and migraine without aura. However, three genes for familial hemiplegic migraine, a rare type of migraine with aura characterized by paralysis on one side of the body, have been identified (CACNA1A, ATP1A2, and SCN1A). While study is ongoing, researchers believe these genes are associated with the spreading cortical depression that may be the cause of migraine aura (see Visual Auras on page 12). Two of these genes have also been linked to epilepsy, which is one of the comorbidities (or associated disorders) of migraine.

 Question

I get migraines. Will my daughter have them?
Family history is a strong risk factor for migraine. But that doesn't necessarily mean your daughter will develop them. Watch for the symptoms of migraine in your child, and consult with a pediatric neurologist if your child begins to complain of head pain. Chapter 12 has more information on children and migraines.

Environmental Factors

There are also a host of factors—including weather, food, stress, hormones, and sleep—that can trigger a migraine attack or episode in migraineurs. These migraine triggers are different from the risk factors described in the previous sections, and they are described in detail in Chapter 6.

There is some evidence that socioeconomic status may also influence the prevalence of migraine. The AMPP study found that adolescents from low-income families with no history of migraine were more likely to develop migraine than those teens from households with an income of $90,000 or higher. However, among those who did have a family history of migraine, there was no difference in migraine prevalence between low-income and higher-income households.

Studies of adult migraineurs have also found that low income is associated with higher migraine prevalence. This seems to indicate that environmental factors associated with low socioeconomic status, such as lack of access to health care, poor diet, and greater levels of stress, may potentially increase migraine risk. It's also possible that chronic migraines—which cause impaired productivity and lost hours in the workplace—may impact the potential for career and wage advancement. Further research is needed to determine the direct relationship between socioeconomic class and migraine.

All about Auras

Auras are associated with changes in blood flow and nerve activity in the brain. They typically last more than five but less than sixty minutes and signal the approach of the migraine headache. Only about one-fifth of the migraine population experiences aura. Bright visual disturbances that spread across the field of vision are the most frequent type of aura reported. Hippocrates described the "shining light" of visual aura as early as 400 B.C.

Visual Auras

Visual disturbance is often the first sign of migraine in many people, and it is the most common type of aura symptom. It may be gradual, building until the sufferer has trouble focusing on a book or computer screen. Or it may be sudden and hit without warning.

In many migraineurs, visual aura appears in the form of flashing lights (*photopsia*). It can also cause visual distortion, blurring, and blind spots (*scotoma*).

A curved, zigzagged band of flashing light that is known clinically as *teichopsia* or a *fortification spectrum* because of its resemblance to the design of a fort wall, may be seen in classic migraine. It often sits on the margin of a crescent-shaped blind spot and grows and moves across the visual field as the aura progresses. These auras can be as brief as five minutes or as long as an hour, but usually peak around twenty minutes after the first visual sign. On average, visual auras last fifteen to twenty minutes.

Blood flow and magnetic resonance imaging (MRI) have shown that during a visual aura, changes take place in the cerebral cortex—the part of the brain that is responsible for thought, memory, and cognition. Blood flow to this part of the brain is reduced, while the activity of the neurons—the nerve cells that transmit and receive electrical and chemical signals across the brain—are suppressed. That suppression spreads across the cortex at a rate of three to six millimeters a minute, which correlates with the rate at which the aura travels across the visual field. This phenomenon is known clinically as *spreading cortical depression.*

 Alert

Visual disturbances that last three to ten minutes, involve a darkening or dimming of vision, and rapidly move across the visual field from the bottom up or from top to bottom, like a shade, may be signs of a transient ischemic attack (TIA), or ministroke, and require immediate medical attention.

Nonvisual Characteristics of Auras

Spreading cortical depression can be associated with the mild speech problems (called *dysphasia*) and one-sided tingling or numbing sensation in an arm or leg (called *paresthesia*) during an aura. Other nonvisual characteristics of aura include dizziness, weakness, and occasionally, nausea.

Migraine Myths and Misconceptions

As previously noted, there is abundant misinformation about the causes and treatment of migraines in the general population and, in some cases, among health care professionals. If you or someone you love live with migraine, it's important to separate fact from fiction and educate those around you who seem convinced of some of the more common misconceptions about this disease.

Learn how to debunk the following common migraine myths:

- **"It's just a headache."** It's easy for those who have never experienced the pain and disability caused by migraine disease to trivialize the disorder. But migraine is not "just a headache." It's a neurological disorder that can impact your ability to work, go to school, and enjoy life—especially if your migraines are frequent.
- **"Sure, it hurts, but I just have to deal with it."** The head pain of migraine is not something you have to suffer through. By getting a proper diagnosis and working with your health care provider, you can find the treatment option that's right for you.
- **"My chronic headaches can't be migraines, because they only happen when I'm stressed."** Stress is a common trigger for a migraine attack. Many people believe that because their head pain is triggered by stress, they must have a tension headache. Migraines are usually focused on one side of the head, while the pain of tension headache is usually described as a tight band around the head. A full diagnostic work up by your health care provider can help you determine what type of headache you have.
- **"Migraine is a symptom of mental health issues."** While some mental disorders, such as depression and anxiety disorder, occur more commonly in migraineurs, they are not the cause of migraine and not everyone with migraine experiences these conditions. Furthermore, it's unclear whether the association is the result of living with chronic migraine pain

or if it's truly a comorbid condition. Depression and anxiety are certainly valid reactions to dealing with chronic migraine pain.

- **"I'm still able to function, so it must not be a migraine."** Migraine pain may be moderate to severe. If you're just getting by when you suffer a migraine attack, remember that there are many treatment options available to you that can improve your quality of life tremendously.

- **"Most people who have migraines are just hypochondriacs."** Migraine has a clear diagnostic framework. Neurological imaging studies show visible changes in the brain during a migraine attack. Specific genes have been linked to some types of migraine. It is a medical disorder that has been documented extensively in the medical literature, and the physical, emotional, and financial toll migraine takes is very real.

CHAPTER 2

When It's *Not* a Migraine

WHILE A MIGRAINE is perhaps the most well-known headache type, not all chronic head pain is migraine. Often, headache is a symptom of an underlying medical condition. Sinus problems, vision disorders, cardiovascular disease, infections, and certain neurological issues may cause frequent headache and in some cases may mimic migraine. There are also several other headache types, such as cluster headaches and tension headaches, which can cause persistent head pain that is just as debilitating as migraine.

Cluster Headaches
Intense and often excruciating unilateral pain that is accompanied by one-sided facial symptoms such as flushing, congestion, and swollen eye, may be cluster headache. The pain is described as stabbing or knifelike, and it radiates toward the eye or jaw from the temple.

The name "cluster headache" comes from the frequency and course of the condition. These headaches occur in distinct patterns of close and frequent attacks, or clusters, recurring over two weeks to three months, followed by headache-free "remission" periods that can last anywhere from a month to several years. About half of cluster headache sufferers experience a headache daily during a cluster episode, and an estimated 33 percent experience two or more headaches in a twenty-four-hour period. The headaches themselves often occur at the same time each day and last fifteen minutes to three hours, with an average headache duration of forty-five minutes. Many experience headache waking them one to two hours after falling asleep.

Cluster headache attacks that occur in episodes of one week to a year, but are separated by a remission period of a month or longer, are called *episodic cluster headache*. Some people with episodic cluster headache may only experience one attack a year, at the same time each year. However, for between 10 and 15 percent of cluster headache sufferers, the condition is chronic—meaning that they have cluster attacks that last longer than a year with no remission, or they experience remission periods of less than one month.

Unlike most headache disorders, cluster headache occurs more frequently in men than in women. Men are three to four times more likely to develop cluster headaches, and the condition typically makes its first appearance between the ages of twenty and forty years old. Cluster headache is relatively rare, impacting less than 1 of every 1,000 adults, according to the World Health Organization.

Making the Diagnosis

Cluster headache is one of a group of headache types known clinically as trigeminal autonomic cephalgias, or TACs. These headaches involve the trigeminal nerve (fifth cranial nerve), the largest nerve of the head that is the gatekeeper for the nerve conduction that supplies sensation to the face. No one knows for sure what triggers the pain of cluster headache. It may be caused by a disorder of the brain's pacemakers, and recent observations suggest that there are abnormalities in the structure and connections in the part of the brain called the hypothalamus in individuals who suffer with this condition. This region of the brain is also responsible for many of the body's autonomic, or involuntary, nervous system functions, and so it is not surprising that these headaches are accompanied by a chain reaction of autonomic responses including facial flushing, tearing of the eye, and drooping of the eyelid.

Sometimes, an undiagnosed cluster headache sufferer will seek help for the facial symptoms of the disorder. A dentist or ear-nose-throat (ENT) specialist may be consulted about recurring tooth, jaw, and/or sinus pain.

Because the pain of cluster headache is on one side of the head, it can be misdiagnosed as migraine. The severity and the pattern of the headache pain can help distinguish cluster headache from migraine. In addition, cluster headache can cause a general sense of restlessness and agitation, while migraineurs, in contrast, typically feel the need to withdraw and rest in a darkened quiet room.

The International Headache Society (IHS) defines cluster headache as five or more episodes of head pain that meet the following diagnostic criteria:

- Severe or very severe one-sided pain in or above the eye or in the temporal (temple) area of the head that lasts fifteen minutes to three hours (if left untreated)
- The headache is accompanied by at least one of the following symptoms:
  - Swelling and redness and/or tearing of the eye on the same side as the head pain
  - Congestion and/or runny nose on the same side as the head pain
  - Swelling of the eyelid that is on the same side as the head pain
  - Sweating of the face and forehead on the same side as the head pain
  - Constriction of the pupil and/or drooping of the eyelid on the same side as the head pain
  - A sense of restlessness or agitation
- Attacks have a frequency from one every other day to eight per day
- Pain is not attributable to another medical disorder

It's important to note that although the above criteria places a time limit on an untreated headache episode, the IHS also says that up to half of attacks may be of shorter or longer duration, and some of these may also be less severe. In addition, the frequency of attacks (i.e., one every other day to eight per day) in a single headache "cluster," or course, may be lower up to half of the time.

 Fact

> Cluster headache often follows seasonal or time-of-day patterns. For this reason, researchers believe that cluster headache may be caused by abnormalities of the hypothalamus, which regulates our circadian cycles (or internal clock). Positron emission tomography (PET) scans have shown heightened activity in the hypothalamus during a cluster attack.

Triggers

There are a number of known triggers for cluster headaches, and recognizing and avoiding them can help reduce the frequency of cluster episodes. Some triggers occur only during an attack period, and others will bring on a cluster episode after months of remission. For example, drinking alcohol during a remission period may not bother you at all, but having a drink during an active cluster period can cause a sudden cluster headache. And many people with cluster headaches have seasonal triggers for their cluster periods; for example, they may experience a cluster period every autumn.

Researchers have discovered a strong correlation between sleep patterns and cluster headache frequency and recurrence, so if you suffer from cluster headaches it's important to stay on a regular, fixed sleep schedule. Variances, such as an afternoon nap or a late night of studying, can trigger an attack.

Other known cluster headache triggers include:

- Smoking and alcohol
- Nitroglycerin used to treat heart conditions

- Exposure to solvents and gasoline
- Hypoxia (insufficient oxygen) due to sleep apnea or high altitude

Treatment

One of the most effective and safest treatments for cluster headache pain is oxygen therapy. Inhaling 100 percent oxygen delivered at seven liters per minute through a mask can usually provide relief within five to fifteen minutes, with no side effects. However, because of the equipment involved, some patients may find oxygen therapy impractical. And while it is effective in about 90 percent of cluster headache patients, it doesn't work for everyone. And in some cases, head pain returns after the oxygen is discontinued.

Because the head pain of cluster headaches comes on severely and quickly, most over-the-counter analgesics aren't very effective. Medication for cluster headache is often administered via nasal spray or injection for rapid absorption.

Drug therapies for acute cluster headache pain include:

Abortive medications:

- **Sumatriptan (Imitrex):** An effective drug delivered via nasal spray or subcutaneous injection. It's not recommended for people with certain heart problems.
- **Zolmatriptan (Zomig):** A triptan drug available in oral and nasal spray form. Side effects may include dry mouth, dizziness, sweating, and weakness. Zomig should also be avoided in patients with heart conditions.
- **Ergotamine:** Available in injectable, inhaler, and sublingual form. Nausea may be a problem with the use of these medications, which can also be dangerous if used more frequently than prescribed.
- **Intranasal lidocaine:** This topical pain reliever is delivered in nasal drops or spray. It can decrease pain within five minutes and abort a headache within thirty-five minutes but is not consistently effective.

- **Intranasal capsaicin:** Also applied to the inside of the nasal cavity, capsaicin has been shown to reduce headache severity after a week of treatment.

Prophylactic, or preventative, therapies are used for chronic or episodic cluster headache. These include:

Prophylactic medications:

- **Verapamil:** An oral drug usually taken three times daily or once daily in a sustained-release preparation that can reduce the frequency of cluster attacks. A common side effect is constipation.
- **Prednisone:** An oral steroid usually prescribed along with another prophylactic. Prednisone works quickly to prevent cluster headache, but because the adverse side effects of the drug start to increase with the length of time it is taken, prednisone is usually used temporarily while another prophylactic medication works its way up to therapeutic levels.
- **Ergotamine derivatives:** A fast-acting drug available in a tablet that dissolves under the tongue and is taken thirty to sixty minutes before an anticipated attack. Ergotamine derivatives can be particularly helpful for patients who experience cluster attacks during sleep. These drugs cannot be used in conjunction with triptans.
- **Lithium:** Effective in cluster prevention, but patients can become resistant to the drug over time. Long-term use and excessive dosing can produce tremor and can cause damage to the kidneys and thyroid, so frequent blood tests are required.
- **Valproic acid (Depakote):** Usually helps prevent attacks within four days after starting treatment. Frequent blood and liver function tests are required for patients taking this therapy.

In patients not responsive to oxygen or drug therapy, an anesthetic nerve block injected into the occipital nerve may be attempted for pain relief. Surgical options involving manipulation or destruction of a portion of the facial nerves are also available, but due to the high risk of permanent nerve damage, these are a last-resort treatment.

Tension Headaches

Tension-type headache (TTH) is the most common type of primary headache, with up to 78 percent of the general population experiencing a headache episode in their lifetime. An estimated 38 percent of people with TTH have experienced a headache within the past year, and studies suggest that most people with TTH experience headache once or twice each month and describe the head pain as moderate in intensity. Like migraine, TTH is more common in women than in men.

The pain of a tension-type headache is often described as a tight band encircling the top of the head, mild to moderate in severity. It differs from migraine and cluster headache in that it is felt on both sides of the head and there is no nausea involved. While a TTH may infrequently cause hypersensitivity to light or sound, as a migraine does, only one of these symptoms usually occurs (not both together as happens frequently with migraine).

A TTH lasts from thirty minutes to seven days and has at least two of the following characteristics:

- Bilateral (both sides of the head)
- Pain is tightness or pressure ("viselike"), not pulsating
- Mild to moderate intensity
- Not made worse by routine physical activity

In some cases, the head may be tender to the touch (called pericranial tenderness). Pain may be felt in the back of the neck and at the base of the skull. The headache itself may cause sleep problems, irritability, difficulty concentrating, and fatigue.

If tension-type headaches are occurring for fewer than fifteen days a month, they are considered episodic tension-type headaches. When tension-type headaches last for hours and are continuous during fifteen or more days of the month for a period of longer than three months, they are considered chronic tension-type headaches.

 Fact

A large U.S. study published in the *Journal of the American Medical Association* found that men and women with higher levels of education were more likely to experience tension-type headache. The opposite trend has been found in migraine, where lower socioeconomic levels seem to be linked to higher migraine occurrence.

Triggers and Treatment

A headache diary can be useful in diagnosing tension-type headache and in identifying headache trends and triggers (see Appendix B for a sample headache diary). Triggers for TTH can include:

- Stress and anxiety
- Sleep problems
- Poor posture
- Fasting or skipping meals
- Overuse of certain medications (e.g., analgesics, cold medications)
- Hormonal changes
- Teeth grinding (bruxism)

In addition, TTH can be a symptom of an underlying medical condition. Dental problems, depression, temporomandibular joint dysfunction (TMJ), respiratory tract infections, hypothyroidism, arthritis, and allergies can all be associated with tension-type headache. In most cases, appropriate treatment of the medical condition can resolve tension-type headaches.

Treatment

Over-the-counter (OTC) pain relievers such as aspirin, ibuprofen (Motrin, Advil), naproxen sodium (Aleve), and acetaminophen (Tylenol) are all very effective in treating occasional and episodic tension-type headaches. Analgesics combined with caffeine (Excedrin), which constricts blood vessels, may also be useful. When TTH doesn't respond to OTC analgesics, prescription pain relievers may be used.

 Alert

OTC and prescription pain relievers should be used in the minimum dosage no more than twice a week to avoid what is known as "rebound headache," or headache caused by medication overuse. Chronic overuse of these drugs can also cause serious gastrointestinal problems and liver damage.

Some studies have also indicated that acupuncture and biofeedback may be useful in relieving TTH pain. Lifestyle changes are also encouraged to help prevent tension-type headache episodes. Because sedentary lifestyle is a risk factor for developing TTH, starting an exercise routine can help. So can healthy sleep and nutrition habits and stress management and relaxation techniques.

Sinus/Nasal Problems

Allergies, infections, and the common cold can all cause swelling and pressure to build up in the sinus cavity that can lead to what is sometimes called a "sinus headache." This inflammation is called sinusitis, and it can cause persistent head pain under the eyes and at the cheekbone, sometimes extending down into the top half of the mouth. Sinus headache may be one-sided or occur on both sides of the face. The sinus may also be obstructed by pus or mucus, causing further pressure and pain. Head pain associated with these conditions can be severe, but fortunately, severe head pain should not accompany the most common forms of upper airway congestion. Nonetheless, common misconceptions about the nature of these conditions by headache sufferers and physicians alike often lead to the misdiagnosis of migraine as sinusitis.

In the short term, a sinus headache can be relieved with over-the-counter analgesic drugs (Tylenol, Aleve, Motrin), but if an infection is present, it should be treated with antibiotics. Sinusitis caused by allergies may require an antihistamine. A decongestant can help relieve sinus pressure, and moist air from a warm shower, vaporizer, or humidifier can help clear sinus cavities.

Essential

To relieve sinus headache pain, the American Academy of Otolaryngology recommends alternating hot and cold compresses on the sinus area of the face. The hot compress should be applied for three minutes, followed by twenty seconds for the cold compress. This procedure should be repeated three times per treatment, two to six times daily.

Sometimes, a structural problem within the sinus and/or nasal cavities can cause pressure and head pain. These may include:

- Malformations of the turbinate bones of the nasal cavity
- Polyps obstructing the sinuses
- Deviated septum

In these cases, surgery may be required to resolve the symptoms.

Central Nervous System Disorders

Once diagnosed, most chronic head pain is treatable with medication and/or lifestyle changes. But rarely, head pain is a symptom of a serious neurological problem, especially if it comes on suddenly and severely without a prior headache history. Inflammation of the nerves or blood vessels connected to the brain, hemorrhage in or around the brain, changes in cerebrospinal fluid (CSF) pressure, development of a brain lesion or mass (either benign or malignant), head injury, and central nervous system infection can all produce headache.

Other neurological disorders and diseases that have headache as a symptom include multiple sclerosis, trigeminal neuralgia, and pseudo-tumor cerebri (also known as idiopathic intracranial hypertension).

Essential

Remember, brain tumors are extremely rare—affecting only 7 in 100,000 people, in the U.S. population each year. Most head pain is caused by more benign, and easily treatable, health conditions.

Brain Tumor

Only 8 percent of patients with brain tumor have headache as a first symptom, but up to 70 percent of diagnosed brain tumor patients will eventually experience regular headache as a symptom. Headache is usually associated with increased intracranial pressure caused by the tumor mass, but head pain may be mild in the case of a slow-growing tumor. Sometimes these headaches are at their worst in the morning and lessen in intensity throughout the day. They are frequently accompanied by nausea and vomiting, and they may get worse when bending over or coughing.

When It's an Emergency

Sometimes, severe head pain that comes on rapidly and without warning is a sign of a medical crisis. Headache is a defining feature of several brain and cardiovascular emergencies, including stroke, meningitis, and subarachnoid hemorrhage.

Red flags for headache emergencies include:

- A headache that develops suddenly and dramatically in a person with no prior headache history

- Severe and sudden headache that is different from normal headache symptoms in someone with a history of headache
- A "thunderclap" headache—a sudden and severe headache that appears without warning and might be described as "the worst headache you've ever had"
- Headache accompanied by fever and/or neck stiffness (which could point to meningitis)
- Headache accompanied by neurological signs such as vertigo, visual disturbance, speech difficulty, and balance problems

Cardiovascular Disorders

The heart and blood vessels keep the nerve pathways of the brain and central nervous system supplied with oxygen-rich blood. When those vessels become blocked, inflamed, or damaged, they can cut off this blood supply and permanently damage nerve fibers and cause infarction, or death, of brain tissue. In people with a history of heart and circulatory problems, sudden or severe head pain can be a sign of more serious problems and should be immediately evaluated by a physician or emergency health care professional.

Circulatory Problems

People with cerebral arteriosclerosis frequently experience headache. Arteriosclerosis occurs when the artery walls thicken and become inflexible. If this occurs in the cerebral blood vessels, it restricts blood flow and can cut off the oxygen supply to the brain, resulting in a stroke. It can also increase the risk of an aneurysm, a weakened blood vessel wall that may be distended and is in danger of rupture, causing hemorrhage, or bleeding on the brain.

Severe and sudden headache is a warning sign of aneurysm and should be evaluated by a medical professional as soon as possible.

Cerebral venous sinus thrombosis, or the formation of clots within the large draining veins of the brain, can also trigger severe head pain. This is a rare disorder associated with conditions that cause hypercoagulability, or excessive clotting, of the blood. These conditions include certain genetic traits, dehydration, infection, contraceptives, and the immediate postpartum period.

A dissection, or tear, in the inner wall of the carotid artery, the major blood vessel located in your neck, causes blood to leak into the artery wall, resulting in head and neck pain. Carotid dissection can also cause a transient ischemic attack (TIA) or a stroke, as the carotid artery narrows and diminishes the blood supply to the brain.

Certain drugs prescribed to treat cardiovascular disease, including blood pressure medications (antihypertensives and vasodilators), may also cause headaches in some people. If your blood pressure medication is causing chronic headache, talk to your doctor about a dosage adjustments and other treatment alternatives.

 Alert

Be aware of the warning signs of stroke: weakness and numbness (often on one side of the body), mental confusion, difficulty speaking, balance problems, vision loss, and a sudden and severe headache. Receiving "clot busting" drugs within three hours after the first signs of a stroke reduces long-term disability in stroke patients.

Transient Ischemic Attack and Stroke

When blood flow to the brain is reduced, a transient ischemic attack, or "ministroke," can occur. The warning signs of TIA are the same as those of stroke—weakness, numbness, confusion, vision loss, difficulty speaking, severe headache—except they disappear in minutes to hours. Because all of these are also found in migraine, there is a possibility of misdiagnosing TIA as migraine or vice versa. If symptoms come on gradually, migraine is the most likely explanation, especially in young people. If head pain and other symptoms are sudden, with maximal severity within seconds to just minutes, TIA or stroke must be considered.

TIA is usually caused by a blockage in the carotid artery or in the smaller blood vessels of the brain that restricts blood flow. This can be due to clotting or to narrowing of the arterial walls. An estimated 20 percent of people who experience a TIA have a stroke within two years. Aspirin and other antiplatelet drugs, anticoagulant drugs (blood thinners) in the setting of certain associated conditions of the heart or blood vessels, surgery to open clogged blood vessels, angioplasty and stents (a wire mesh tube that holds the artery open) can also reduce the risk of TIA and stroke.

 Fact

When compared to those without migraine, men with migraine disorder have an increased risk for cardiovascular disease and heart attack. Among women, those who have migraine with aura are at an increased risk for cardiovascular disease, heart attack, transient ischemic attack, and stroke.

Vision Problems

Refractive errors—or problems with the focusing of light by the eye—can be the cause of persistent tension-type headache. Uncorrected refractive errors cause problems with visual acuity, making things blurry and unfocused. As your eyes attempt to compensate for the vision deficit, forehead and scalp muscles contract excessively, especially with squinting, and headache can result. And because the focusing ability of the eye decreases with age, the problem becomes more common as you grow older. The good news is that this type of headache is usually easily corrected with glasses, contact lenses, or corrective laser surgery.

Eyestrain, or asthenopia, can also cause a dull, frontal headache. People who work at computer screens for long periods of time or do a lot of "close work" often experience this type of visual fatigue. Sometimes this is associated with uncorrected refractive errors. Rest and properly prescribed eyeglasses are often helpful.

Diseases of the Optic Nerve

The optic nerve connects the back of the eye to the brain and is responsible for transmitting visual images in the form of nerve impulses from the retina to the brain. When the nerve is damaged by pressure or inflammation, vision distortion and/or loss can occur. Headache, especially in the region of the affected eye is a frequent symptom of diseases of the optic nerve.

Glaucoma is a visual disorder characterized by optic nerve damage resulting from elevated pressure within the eye that can result in partial to complete vision loss. Both headache and eye pain are warning signs of severe elevation of eye pressure and are an indication for immediate treatment by an ophthalmologist.

Retrobulbar optic neuritis is caused by inflammation of the optic nerve. The condition can be caused by viral infections and has a strong association with multiple sclerosis, a disease of the central nervous system. Head pain focused around the eye is a common feature, especially at the extremes of movement of the eye within the eye socket.

Other Migraine Mimickers

As you've learned, headache is caused by a wide variety of environmental and physical factors. And when chronic head pain resembles the vascular, pulsating headache of migraine, it can be difficult for both doctors and patients to distinguish between the two.

Following are some causes of vascular headache that can be mistaken for migraine:

- **Viral and bacterial infections**. Many infections and illnesses, especially those associated with fever—such as pneumonia, mumps, measles, flu, chicken pox, salmonella, and Lyme disease—have associated headache.
- **Caffeine withdrawal**. Caffeine is actually used in some migraine treatments to help relieve migraine pain. But if you overdo your caffeine intake, cutting back or going cold turkey can result in a pounding vascular headache.

- **Lumbar puncture.** This medical procedure, in which a needle is inserted into the spinal canal to remove a small amount of cerebrospinal fluid (CSF), can cause a change in CSF pressure that triggers what is known as a lumbar puncture headache. Like a migraine, the headache is frequently accompanied by nausea and vomiting, but easily distinguishing it from migraine is the sharp worsening upon standing and rapid relief upon lying down. A lumbar puncture headache caused by continued leaking of CSF from the puncture site can be easily treated with a blood patch—an injection of the patient's blood into the epidural space to create a blood clot over the puncture hole.
- **Nitrates and nitrites.** Nitrates are drugs prescribed to patients with angina and congestive heart failure. They dilate, or open, the blood vessels, which can cause vascular headache and facial flushing in some people. A similar compound, sodium nitrite, is used as a preservative in many processed meats, including hot dogs and lunchmeat. Look for sodium nitrite or nitrate on food labels to identify nitrites.
- **Temporal arteritis.** Also called giant cell arteritis, temporal arteritis is caused by chronic inflammation of the large vessels that supply blood to the face and scalp, branches of the external carotid artery. The condition is most frequently found in adults over age fifty. Because the main symptom is a pulsating headache associated with visual disturbances, it may be misdiagnosed as migraine. This is a potentially serious condition, and prompt treatment with corticosteroids is required to reduce inflammation and prevent vision loss.

Headache can be caused by literally hundreds of medical conditions and environmental factors, from hangover to head injury. Seeing a qualified medical health care professional and keeping a written record of your symptoms is the best way to get an accurate diagnosis of the cause of your head pain.

CHAPTER 3

Diagnosis

PROPER DIAGNOSIS OF head pain is the first step in getting your migraines under control. If your primary care doctor is not experienced in headache evaluation and treatment, he may refer you to a headache specialist or neurologist. In order to diagnose your head pain, your provider will take a medical history, perform a physical and neurological examination, and order appropriate tests. He may also administer assessments, or short questionnaires, designed to help evaluate the nature of your headaches and the impact they have on your daily life.

Keeping a Headache Diary

A headache diary is a journal of when your headaches occur, the circumstances surrounding them, and the symptoms you experience before, during, and after a headache episode. By tracking your headaches in this way, you provide your doctor with information that will be invaluable in diagnosing what type of primary headache you have (migraine or otherwise).

Headache diaries are also important for gathering information on those things that might trigger a headache attack, such as certain foods, stress, lighting, weather changes, and other environmental factors. They can also help you identify any symptoms that consistently precede an attack. If possible, start a diary prior to your first doctor's appointment. It will help your provider take a more accurate medical history.

Diary Basics

When you document your headaches, try to note your activities prior to the headache episode, including what you ate, physical activity, sleep patterns, exposure to any unusual odors or visual stimuli (i.e., bright lights, high contrast patterns), notable changes in weather, and emotional stress.

For premenopausal women, it's also important to note where you are in your menstrual cycle when your headaches occur because migraines are often associated with hormonal changes.

Tracking Treatments

Keep track of any medications you take as well, including vitamins, supplements, and over-the-counter drugs. Some medications can cause headache, including overuse of certain pain relievers. If environmental factors such as temperature, lighting, and changes in humidity ease your head pain, note this as well. Also note those environmental changes that make your head pain worse.

Chapter 5 covers headache diaries in further detail. You can also find a sample headache diary in Appendix B.

Screening Assessments

Screening assessments, also called measures, tools, and tests, are questions your doctor will ask in order to determine if you have migraine and to gauge the impact migraine is having on your quality of life. Assessments may be a short series of simple questions your doctor asks during your office visit, or they may be longer written evaluations.

Is It a Migraine?

ID Migraine is a three-question screening tool that identifies headache-related nausea, photophobia (light sensitivity), and disability. It is one of the few screening assessments that has been validated for high sensitivity in clinical trials. And because it's very quick and specific, in addition to being highly accurate, it's a good tool for both patients and physicians. ID Migraine consists of these questions:

- Has a headache limited your activities for a day or more in the last three months?
- Are you nauseated or sick to your stomach when you have a headache?
- Does light bother you when you have a headache?

Patients who answer yes to at least two out of the three questions are identified as likely migraineurs who should undergo a further diagnostic workup. There is also a longer, nine-item version of the assessment that your doctor may use.

Functional and Quality-of-Life Assessments

The Functional Assessment in Migraine (FAIM) questionnaire is a screening tool that assesses how migraine affects your physical and mental functioning during an attack. FAIM includes subscales that are used to determine how migraine impacts work productivity and participation in day-to-day activities.

There are a number of patient assessment tools your doctor may use to measure the impact that migraine has on your quality of life and the level of disability caused by the condition. These include:

- **The Headache Impact Test (HIT):** A written six-item test that measures the impact headaches have on daily functioning at home, work, school, and in social situations. There is also an online version of this assessment.
- **The Migraine Disability Assessment (MIDAS):** A seven-item written questionnaire designed to assess migraine-related disability.
- **Migraine Specific Quality of Life Survey (MSQ or MSQoL):** A twenty-item assessment to assess quality of life in migraineurs.

- **Headache Needs Assessment Questionnaire (HANA):** A fourteen-question assessment of the frequency and "bothersomeness" of chronic head pain.

Medical History and Physical Exam

Your doctor will want to quickly establish whether your headaches have a primary or secondary cause by reviewing your medical history and conducting a full physical examination. Secondary headaches are headaches that are symptomatic of another medical condition (see Chapter 2). Headaches that have a sudden and severe onset can indicate a serious medical condition, such as stroke or meningitis, so establishing the nature of this type of head pain is critical. Migraines are a primary type of headache.

By reviewing and updating your medical history, your doctor may be able to determine if any preexisting medical conditions or current medications could be at the root of your headaches. Your doctor will also ask you about any history of headaches in your family.

L., Essential

If you're brand new to a physician's practice, you should arrange to have your previous medical records and any lab or radiological test results sent over prior to your visit. If they aren't available, your provider should take a full medical history at your first appointment.

Medical History

Your doctor will probably start with an assessment of the reason you're there—your headaches. She will want to know about the location, severity, frequency, and nature of the head pain, and any other symptoms that occur along with it, such as visual changes or nausea. She will also ask about what makes the pain lessen, what makes it feel worse, whether you have tried medication and comfort measures like compresses, and how successful they've been. It's also important for your doctor to evaluate what impact your headaches are having on your everyday functioning, quality of life, and emotional well-being. This is where your headache diary comes in handy.

Your medical history should include documentation of any serious past illnesses, infections, allergies, and surgeries, and it should also note family history of any disease. If other doctors are prescribing medications for you, make sure you bring a list of them to your appointment. Try to be precise about the names and dosage of any medication you are taking now and for any medication you have previously taken for your headaches. Your provider will inquire about lifestyle issues that could have an impact on your health, including smoking, sleep and nutrition habits, alcohol and caffeine use, sexual history, sources of stress, and exercise routine.

 Fact

Approximately 67 percent of neurologists have had at least one migraine in their lifetime, and 50 percent are current migraine sufferers. Compare that to a 12 percent lifetime prevalence seen in the general population. Sympathy pains? No. It's more likely this phenomenon is because neurologists are more aware of the symptoms of migraine.

Physical Exam

A full physical examination is also key in establishing the cause and nature of your headaches. It can also reveal underlying causes for secondary head pain. In addition to taking your vital signs (i.e., blood pressure, temperature, pulse rate, and respiratory rate), your doctor will listen to your heart and lungs, examine your skin and extremities, and check for any neck stiffness. She will also conduct a head, eyes, ears, nose, and throat examination (called HEENT in medical shorthand) to establish whether your head pain is caused by a sinus problem. Last but not least is the neurological evaluation, a key part of any physical exam involving headache.

Neurological Evaluation and Workup

A neurological evaluation or examination consists of a series of simple tests that allow your provider to assess your brain and nerve function. Any unusual findings on the neurological evaluation may indicate a need for further diagnostic neurological workup, including computerized tomography (CT) scan or magnetic resonance imaging (MRI). It's important to note that these tests can't confirm a diagnosis of migraine, but they can help to rule out disease-based causes of head pain in patients with daily or almost daily headache pain.

The Neurological Evaluation

A complete neurological exam should include the following:

- **Mental status assessment:** Your doctor will ask you questions to assess speech, memory, comprehension, abstract reasoning, and orientation to environment (i.e., awareness of time and place).
- **Cranial nerve tests:** There are twelve cranial nerves that control vision; hearing; taste; smell; pupil reactivity to light; tongue and lip movement; gag reflex; and sensation in the face, head, and neck. A variety of different exams are used to assess these functions.
- **Motor system:** Assessment of muscle strength and tone. The doctor will also look for any involuntary twitches or tremors.
- **Sensory system:** The use of pain, pressure, temperature, and position to check for loss of sensation. Sensory tests are used on the hands, feet, face, and trunk. The pain test isn't as bad as it sounds; the physician takes a pin and touches it lightly to the skin to determine if you can feel it. Your doctor may also

use a blunt object to trace letters or numbers onto your palm and ask you to identify them.

- **Deep tendon reflexes:** This is the familiar rubber hammer reflex test. The hammer triggers nerve stimulation that causes muscles to contract, causing involuntary movement. If the movement doesn't occur, it indicates a signaling problem in the nerve pathways.
- **Coordination:** Coordination tests may include alternately touching one's nose and a fixed object; tapping fingers and/ or toes together in a specific pattern; or touching the heel of one foot to the opposite knee and running it down and then back up the shin. These tests can reveal signaling problems in the coordination pathways of the brain.
- **Gait:** Gait is an assessment of your walking stance and step. Walking actually requires a fairly complex integration of brain and muscle signals, so it is a good tool to uncover neurological problems. Your doctor may ask you to walk in a number of different ways, including toe-to-heel, toe walking, or completing a series of turns, and will assess your stance, posture, and balance as you walk.

 Fact

Your neurological exam may include a check for plantar reflex. In this test, the doctor firmly strokes the sole of the foot from heel to ball, which should cause the toes to flex or curl downward. If the toes separate and extend out instead, this is called a positive Babinski sign, and it could indicate some form of a brain or spinal cord problem.

Neuroimaging

Neuroimaging is the technique of imaging, or taking pictures of, the structure and function of the brain and spinal column. Neuroimaging tools include CT scans, which use a series of X-rays compiled by computers to create pictures of cross-sections of the body; and MRI, which uses powerful magnets and radiofrequency waves to create detailed images of almost any region of the body.

Most patients with suspected migraine will not require neuroimaging studies such as CT scan or MRI, but in some cases, these tests may be appropriate. The American Academy of Neurology (AAN) and the U.S. Headache Consortium have developed physician guidelines for ordering neurological imaging studies in headache patients. These guidelines suggest that neuroimaging should be ordered in the following circumstances:

- When a patient has an abnormal finding on a neurological examination (described above).
- When a patient's chronic headache does not neatly fit the diagnostic criteria for a primary headache disorder such as migraine, cluster headache, or tension-type headache.
- When the patient is at a higher risk of a pathological, or disease-based, neurological cause of secondary headache due to family or medical history.
- When clinical "red flags" are present, including a headache that awakens the patient from sleep, abrupt onset of severe headache, abnormal vital signs (e.g., fever, high blood pressure), headache following head trauma, new onset headache in patients under five or over fifty, or headaches triggered by exertion.

In the end, a physician will use his clinical judgment in ordering any neuroimaging studies. Some doctors may order neuroimaging if a patient is extremely fearful or anxious that there may be a pathological, or disease-based cause of their head pain (e.g., brain tumor or cancer) and this fear and anxiety is causing significant distress or disability.

Magnetic Resonance Imaging

An MRI can't diagnose migraine, but it can rule out brain tumor, infection, stroke, and other causes of secondary headache. An MRI may be very helpful if you have any risk factors or red flags of a non-migrainous condition.

MRI is also extremely useful in clinical research on headache and migraine. Studies have shown that migraineurs are more likely to show white matter abnormalities on MRI. Researchers have also used functional magnetic resonance imaging techniques to establish that the aura of migraine is caused by a phenomenon called cortical spreading depression (a unique depression of the metabolic function that seems to migrate over the cortex of the brain).

 Question

Are PET scans useful for migraine diagnosis?
Positron emission tomography (PET) is a nuclear medicine scan that can be used to evaluate metabolic functioning of the brain. It is not useful for migraine diagnosis, but PET scans are used frequently in migraine research and have shown that migraine is associated with specific changes in certain brain regions, especially the brainstem.

Computerized Axial Tomography Scans

A CT scan may be ordered if your provider believes that your headaches may be associated with sinus problems, or if bleeding, swelling, or infection of the brain is suspected. CT scans are also frequently used in patients who show up in urgent care or emergency rooms with sudden severe "thunderclap" headaches because they are more sensitive than MRI in detecting brain hemorrhage. Contrast medium, an iodine-based dye that is injected into the bloodstream to enhance CT images, may be used in a scan.

Alert

If you are allergic to iodine or shellfish; have kidney disease, asthma, heart disease, or multiple myeloma; or take the type 2 diabetes drug metformin (or a combination drug containing metformin), inform your doctor before undergoing any neuroimaging test involving contrast medium.

Lab Tests

As is the case with neuroimaging, there are no currently available lab tests that can diagnose migraine headaches. There are, however, a number of tests that may be ordered by your doctor in order to exclude other causes of headache.

Essential

Certain migraine drugs, including topiramate (Topamax) and divalproex sodium (Depakote) can impact your blood counts and/or blood chemistry. You may require regular blood tests while on these drugs. Ask your doctor if your migraine medication requires you to get regular blood testing.

Blood and Urine Tests

Blood and urine tests can rule out infection and certain disease-based causes of chronic headache such as temporal arteritis, thyroid disease, kidney failure, and anemia. Blood tests may include a complete blood count (CBC), a comprehensive metabolic panel (CMP), and other blood chemistry panels.

A high white blood cell count indicates infection, while a low red cell count points to anemia, both potential causes of secondary headache. An elevated erythrocyte sedimentation rate (sometimes called a sed rate) may mean that the head pain is caused by temporal arteritis.

Other Lab Tests

Infections such as meningitis and conditions causing bleeding on the brain can cause severe headache. A lumbar puncture, also known as a spinal tap, is a procedure that involves removing cerebrospinal fluid (or CSF) from the base of the spine in order to examine the fluid for infection or blood. It is not useful in migraine diagnosis, but lumbar puncture may be used to rule out a subarachnoid hemorrhage if neuroimaging is normal but other factors point to potential bleeding. The procedure is also used to assess CSF pressure when increased intracranial pressure (or swelling of the brain) is suspected.

Putting It All Together

Once your provider has taken your medical history, examined your headache diary, completed the physical and neurological exam, and received the results of any lab or neuroimaging tests, she should have the data needed to make at least a tentative diagnosis of your head pain.

Doctors experienced with headache care are familiar with the International Headache Society diagnostic criteria for migraine, discussed in more detail in Chapter 1. If a patient fits either of the sets of diagnostic criteria and has a normal neurological exam and no other risk factors, but has not yet had five headache episodes, the patient is typically diagnosed with "probable" migraine or migraine with aura.

CHAPTER 4

Getting Help

PROPER DIAGNOSIS OF head pain is just the first step in getting your migraines under control. To uncover headache triggers and determine the most effective course of migraine treatment, you need to find a physician who is experienced in headache medicine and will act as a collaborative partner in care. The right doctor will also work with you to develop an action plan for migraine emergencies, so when you have a migraine crisis and your health care provider is unavailable, you'll know just what to do.

Finding a Doctor

If you have a primary care provider (PCP) that you are happy with, it makes sense to see him for an initial consultation. During the visit you can assess your provider's level of expertise in managing your particular headache situation and determine whether or not he's the best choice for overseeing your migraine treatment. A good provider will offer a referral to a headache specialist or a neurologist if he's inexperienced with migraine care or believes that the source of your head pain warrants further investigation. Remember—if you aren't satisfied with your provider's level of expertise, you have the right to request a referral to a specialist.

In today's managed-care world, patients often seek their medical care from a rotation of doctors in large physician practices or clinics. Many women with an uncomplicated health history have a regular OB/GYN or OB/GYN practice that provides most of their medical care. If you don't have a trusted primary care provider to turn to, there are several ways to find a physician to evaluate and treat your migraines.

⌐ Essential

Don't be afraid to bring up the topic of specialist care during your initial appointment with your primary care provider. Most general practice and internal medicine physicians provide referrals for their patients on a regular basis, and they won't be offended by a referral request.

Where to Look

Networking is a good place to start to get a reality-based opinion of a doctor. If you have family, friends, or coworkers who suffer from migraine, ask about their experience with their current provider. Consider the source as you evaluate these recommendations. What's important to you in a physician may be a lower priority to others. By asking specific questions about the things that matter to you, such as the doctor's experience with headache patients, you will gather more valuable information than you would if you just inquire whether a friend or family member "likes" their doctor.

A call to your health insurer can usually get you a list of physicians with headache treatment experience in your area. Of course, health insurers often impose restrictions on which care providers you can see for migraine care. In some cases, seeing a specialist will require a referral from your primary care provider. If you're dissatisfied with the choices offered by your insurance plan, you may be able to see an "out of network" provider if you're willing to pay a larger portion of the cost.

Finally, both the American Headache Society and the National Headache Foundation offer physician referral services for migraine treatment. See Appendix A for contact information.

Fact

Look past your PCP when you're seeking a migraine referral. Sometimes, other specialists have greater insights. Dentists see a large percentage of patients with headache, and yours may be an excellent source of referrals. And because of the hormone/ migraine connection in women, your OB/GYN probably also knows a few headache specialists.

What to Look For

Aside from the obvious factors like location, office hours, and insurance considerations, there are certain attributes to look for in a physician who can effectively treat your head pain.

Doctors frequently use what is known as a mnemonic, or a memory device, usually an acronym, to help them remember certain symptoms and features of diseases. In your search for a doctor that will be an effective partner in migraine care, you can use your own mnemonic to ensure that you get the relief you're seeking.

- **R**eachable. Is she reasonably accessible? If you phone with a question, will your doctor or an informed member of her staff return your call within a few hours? How does the practice triage, or prioritize, calls from patients?
- **E**xperienced. Does the doctor have experience diagnosing and treating headache? What is their treatment philosophy?
- **L**istener. Health care is a collaborative process, and a doctor should be a partner in care that takes the time to listen to your concerns and answer questions.
- **I**nnovative. Does your doctor read the latest journals and stay up-to-date on new migraine research and treatments? Is she open-minded and willing to try new things?
- **E**mpathetic. This should be a given, but not all doctors are able to express compassion. Choose a physician who shows

that they care about your well-being through their words and actions.

- **Flexible.** A good physician should be able to recognize when a treatment isn't working and change is required. They should also understand that lifestyle factors such as your economic situation, occupation, and family obligations might limit the potential for success of some treatments and be able to tailor a treatment program that works for you.

As part of your initial consultation, your provider should perform a full medical history (or an update of medical history if you're a current patient), physical exam, and neurological evaluation, as described in Chapter 3. If your physician skips any of these steps or prescribes medication without engaging you in a discussion of possible treatment options, you may want to seek a second opinion.

 Question

Is there any accreditation for migraine doctors that I should look for?
Some migraine specialists may have a Certification of Added Qualification (CAQ) in Headache Management from the National Board of Certification in Headache Management (NBCHM) certifying substantial experience treating headache patients. Neurologists may have further certifications; see below for more information.

When It's Time for a Second Opinion

A second opinion may be warranted if your doctor is hesitant or unwilling to give you an official diagnosis or if you aren't clear on the diagnosis he has provided and follow-up questions haven't helped. Seeking a second opinion may also be a good idea if you just don't feel the diagnosis you've been given is accurate. In this case, a second opinion can provide peace of mind and ensure that you're getting the proper care for the right condition.

Once a diagnosis of migraine is given, a discussion of treatment options and how they may, or may not, work with your lifestyle and personal medical history should take place between you and your doctor. He should also discuss those lifestyle changes that may help lessen the frequency of your migraine attacks. If your doctor hands you a prescription with little or no explanation, or ignores any objections you have to the treatment plan he suggests, then a second opinion is probably a good idea.

 Fact

Less than 20 percent of migraineurs end up seeing a neurologist or other headache medicine specialist, even though studies have shown that most patients who see a specialist report more satisfaction with their headache care.

Unfortunately, while the majority of physicians you will encounter understand that migraine is a neurological condition that can cause severe pain and substantial disability, there are still health care professionals out there who will write off migraine as "just a headache." If you ever get the sense that your doctor is discounting your condition or underestimating the impact it is having on your life, it's time to find another health care provider.

Migraine Specialists

General practice physicians and internists may refer you to a specialist for several reasons. If they suspect an underlying disease-based cause of your migraine symptoms or if you have abnormal findings on a neurological exam, they will typically refer you to a neurologist.

If the migraine treatments they have prescribed for you are not working, or if your headaches are increasing in frequency without substantial relief, they may refer you to a neurologist, a headache medicine specialist, or a pain medicine physician.

You can also ask your doctor for a referral to a specialist if you feel that you aren't getting adequate or appropriate migraine care from your primary care doctor. Do keep in mind that migraine treatment is a process, and rarely does the first prescription or treatment plan a doctor develops work perfectly. It may take several changes in prescription, along with lifestyle changes, to achieve relief. However, if you feel your primary care doctor is not being responsive to your needs or just isn't knowledgeable about headache care, you have the right to request a specialist referral.

Some migraine specialists may be MDs who have special training, substantial experience, and continuing medical education (CME) in headache medicine. They may also have a Certification of Added Qualification in Headache Management from the NBCHM. You can find a listing of doctors with this credential online at *www .primarycarenet.org/nhf/nhf_intro.html*.

Neurologists

A neurologist is frequently the first specialist a general practice physician will send a migraine patient to, especially if the patient has an abnormal neurological exam and requires neuroimaging studies such as MRI or CT scan.

A neurologist is a physician who specializes in diseases and disorders of the central nervous system—including the brain, spinal cord, nerves, and muscles. In addition to earning their MD or DO degree and completing a hospital internship, a neurologist has to have undertaken at least three years of specialty training in an accredited neurology residency program. After residency, the neurologist may then go on to earn board certification from the American Board of Psychiatry and Neurology (ABPN, for medical doctors) or the American Board of Osteopathic Neurologists and Psychiatrists (ABONP, for doctors of osteopathy).

Fact

A doctor who specializes in pain medicine may also be helpful in treating your migraines. Both the American Board of Pain Medicine (ABPM) and the American Academy of Pain Management (AAPM) offer pain practitioners diplomate credentialing.

Some neurologists may also have a board certification specific to headache medicine. The United Council of Neurologic Subspecialties (UCNS) certifies physicians in headache medicine, and the National Board of Certification in Headache Management (NBCHM) also offers a Certification of Added Qualification (CAQ) in Headache Management. Certification requires that physicians have substantial experience treating headache patients. Depending on the certification they are pursuing, they may also need to pass a rigorous exam, participate in conferences devoted to headache medicine, publish research related to headache in a peer-reviewed journal, and complete a certain number of continuing medical education courses each year.

After the neurologist confirms or establishes diagnosis, he or she will recommend a course of treatment. A neurologist is more likely to investigate preventative, or prophylactic, therapies for a migraine patient than to only prescribe acute pain-relief medications.

Headache Clinics

Another option for ongoing migraine care is the headache clinic. Headache clinics take a holistic, or "whole-person," approach to migraine treatment. The professional focus of a headache clinic is usually multidisciplinary, with various pain medicine, neurology, counseling, and mental health professionals on staff. Dietitians, pharmacists, and physical therapists may also lend their expertise as the treatment plan is developed. And some clinics even have professionals that specialize in complementary medicine, such as acupuncturists, affiliated with their programs.

Because they tend to be on the leading edge of migraine care, headache clinics are often involved in research and are involved with patient recruitment for clinical trials for new treatments and therapies. A handful of headache clinics also have inpatient programs for complicated migraine cases, such as patients who have comorbid medical conditions and those who may have developed a dependence on pain medications.

Appendix A contains resources for finding headache specialists and clinics in your area.

Working Together

Long-term and successful migraine treatment is a lot more than just finding the right prescription and taking it as directed. You have to remain aware of your migraine triggers, and in some cases, you may have to make lifestyle changes to reach your treatment goals. You also need to keep track of this information so that when you do see your doctor, he can help you assess what's working and what isn't.

Essential

Ask your prospective doctor if he is a physician member or at least aware of the National Headache Foundation and/or the American Headache Society. These organizations provide professionals with the latest information on headache disorders and support migraine-related clinical research and continuing medical education.

At the same time, your doctor should take the time to carefully consider the data you bring him (in the form of your headache diary) and to answer your questions and concerns. That doesn't mean he's expected to read a thirty-page document at each visit. Be as respectful of his time as he should be of yours. Highlight important information or send your diary in advance of your appointment for review. Talk to your doctor to find a process that works well for both of you.

Follow-up appointments should also be collaborative. Make sure you tell your doctor if your migraines start to increase in frequency or the severity or symptoms of your headaches starts to change. Track your medication use carefully. If you find yourself taking more medication with more headaches and less pain relief, you could be experiencing rebound or medication-overuse headache. And if a medication isn't working because it conflicts with certain lifestyle needs, then your doctor should work with you to find something more appropriate

Help Your Doctor Help You

Be forthcoming with any information that can impact your health and your migraine care. This includes recreational drug use, drinking, and sexual activity. Your doctor can't treat you effectively if he has an edited version of your lifestyle and/or things that may trigger a migraine attack. Most physicians have pretty much "seen it all," and hiding information out of embarrassment or guilt can only hurt you. Remember, the doctor-patient relationship is one that is protected by confidentiality, so being open and honest is the best way to get on the path to better migraine management.

You can also help improve your patient care experience by doing some very basic things. Bring your headache diary to every appointment and show up on time and ready for your appointment. No one likes extended waits at the doctor's office, but patients often don't realize that when they are late for appointments, don't cancel or reschedule appointments, or show up at the doctor's office unprepared (e.g., no insurance card, forgotten lab appointments), they contribute to the overall problem.

When to Call Your Doctor

Immediately phone your doctor if you experience any of the emergency symptoms described in "When to Seek Emergency Care" later in this chapter. Make sure that you tell the receptionist or answering service your specific problem so they can have a member of the clinical staff get on the line or return your call immediately. If it's after hours, leave a message with the answering service and then go to your nearest emergency care facility. Get a family member or friend to drive you (or call 911 if you are incapacitated).

You should also phone your physician if you're trying a new medication and it is absolutely not working for you (i.e., you experience little to no pain relief, your headaches increase in frequency). If your follow-up appointment is within the next day or two and you aren't in the midst of a migraine episode, it probably makes sense to have the discussion face-to-face. But if you have a wait of several weeks or longer, make the call.

 Alert

If you experience a migraine episode that lasts for seventy-two hours or longer (known as *status migrainosus*), and your usual medication is not relieving the pain, call your doctor. Your doctor may prescribe another rescue drug, or he may send you to the emergency room or to urgent care for treatment.

The same goes for a new medication that is causing serious side effects, especially if your doctor didn't mention the side effect when he prescribed the drug. If a drug is causing a skin rash, breathing difficulties, or swelling, it's possible you are allergic to it. Discontinue the drug and phone your doctor immediately to report the problem. If breathing problems are severe, call 911 for emergency assistance. Most side effects are of a milder nature and may include stomach upset, sleepiness, and difficulty concentrating, depending on the drug you're taking. If these side effects are causing significant discomfort, then call your doctor. Frequently, side effects will decrease and even disappear over time, but they may warrant a change in prescription.

When It's an Emergency

Headache accounts for over 2 million emergency-room visits each year in the United States. Over half of migraineurs (54 percent) first consult their doctor about their head pain. But 16 percent initially seek help in an emergency room or urgent care setting. And over 20 percent of diagnosed migraineurs have visited an emergency facility in the past twelve months.

Emergency care is not a substitute for ongoing treatment from your doctor. Urgent care and emergency room visits for migraine should be limited to those situations in which pain is not responding to normal treatment and your provider's office is closed. These facilities are for acute care and can't provide continuous care for a chronic condition like migraine disease.

 Fact

There is no current recommended standard of care for emergency-room treatment of migraine headache. Several studies have demonstrated that migraine remains underdiagnosed and undertreated in emergency care facilities. Time and resource pressures in emergency care settings probably contribute to this problem.

When to Seek Emergency Care

Your headache doctor should be your first line of defense if your migraine treatment isn't working. However, there will be times when your physician simply is not available. Before an emergency situation develops, talk to your doctor about how you should handle severe head pain that doesn't respond to treatment when it occurs after office hours. You should develop a plan that outlines what the on-call physician can do for you and what urgent care facility you will visit should the situation require it. Discuss what kind of signs and symptoms should always warrant emergency treatment.

Always seek emergency care:

- If your head pain has lasted for seventy-two hours or longer without relief from standard treatments (known as *status migrainosus* or intractable migraine)
- If you experience a "thunderclap" headache (an intense head pain in which maximal severity occurs immediately at the onset or within seconds of its appearance)
- If you're experiencing a migraine episode that is different from any other you've had and that is causing severe, unresolved pain
- If you lose consciousness during a migraine episode or experience unresolved vision loss and/or mental confusion
- If your headache is accompanied by fever, rapid heart beat, or high blood pressure
- If you have had a blow to the head within the seventy-two hours prior to the headache episode

Being Prepared for the ER

If you need emergency care, make sure a family member or friend accompanies you to the hospital or urgent care center. Driving with a severe migraine can be dangerous, and it's also good to have someone with you to help keep you comfortable and to advocate for you if you're unable to express yourself clearly. Since you may be foggy from the migraine, your companion can also take down any medical instructions from the attending physician.

Ask your regular doctor to provide you with a one-page sheet of emergency treatment guidelines that specifies your diagnosis, medications, any drug allergies, and suggested pain-relief treatment for migraine episodes that don't respond to your regular preventative or abortive migraine drug regimen. Having this information at hand serves two purposes: it helps the ER staff provide you with quick and effective care, and it establishes that you aren't an addict or drug-seeking patient just trying to get access to narcotics (an unfortunate reality in many emergency care facilities).

It is also helpful to have a separate page of information that contains your health insurance information, diagnosis, and the medications you've taken to treat the current migraine episode. Appendix C contains sample doctor and patient forms for your use.

L, Essential

The American College of Emergency Physicians (ACEP) recommends keeping a file of all insurance information, current medications (both prescription and over-the-counter), drug allergies, and pertinent medical records that you can take with you in the event of a trip to the emergency department.

Remember that emergency departments triage patients, seeing those with the most life-threatening conditions first. It isn't "first come first served." This may mean a substantial wait before you're seen. It doesn't mean that emergency personnel are ignoring you or aren't taking your pain seriously. Most facilities will get you into an exam room where you can rest as soon as the space frees up, even if there is still a long wait ahead until a provider will be available. And they will do their best to make you comfortable in the waiting area.

About Urgent Care

The next time it's after doctor's office hours and you have a severe migraine that just won't respond to treatment, try a local urgent care center instead of the emergency department. A 2006 survey by the National Headache Foundation found that on most measures of migraine patient satisfaction, urgent care centers scored significantly higher than emergency departments. Patients who visited urgent care centers were more likely to be given a quiet place to rest while they waited for treatment, receive care in under an hour, and feel as if the treatment they received was effective.

Urgent care centers are designed as backup facilities for when your doctor is unavailable, and because they are commercial enterprises that want your repeat business and referrals, you may find an overall higher level of "customer service." Any truly life-threatening emergency cases that visit an urgent care center will be sent on to the hospital emergency department, so the long waits involved with triaging the "sickest" patients first are usually minimal.

CHAPTER 5

Headache Diaries

WHEN YOU HAVE a primary headache disorder like migraine, it's very important to track the frequency, length, and characteristics of your headache episodes. Having this information at the time of your initial evaluation will help your health care provider identify specific patterns in your headache progression and be better able to properly diagnose and treat you. A headache diary can also help you and your doctor determine if medications or other treatments are working well for you during your ongoing headache management.

Why Keep a Headache Diary?

A headache diary is an important tool to help you and your doctor figure out what kind of headaches you have and how to avoid the things that cause them. If you've already been diagnosed with migraine and you've started a treatment plan, the diary is also invaluable in evaluating the effectiveness of medication and lifestyle changes. If your headaches hit without warning, you should carry the diary with you at all times. It may take some effort and organization for you to keep on top of your headache diary, but there are strategies you can use to make tracking your headaches easier.

Keeping a headache diary can be as simple as taking notes on a calendar or as complex as entering data into a spreadsheet or computer program. If you carry a date book or organizer with you already, you might use it to track your headache information. Whatever method you choose, make sure it's easy for you so you're more likely to do it. If you're going in for an initial evaluation of your head pain, it's recommended that you keep your headache diary for as long as possible prior to your appointment. But any amount of information will be helpful to your doctor, so don't put off starting your diary if you have less than six weeks until your appointment.

Fact

Studies have shown that using a headache diary for at least three months is highly effective in diagnosing menstrual migraine. Menstrual migraine—or migraine associated with the hormonal fluctuations of the menstrual cycle—affects an estimated 12.6 million American women.

Some people are put off by the idea of a headache diary because they don't like the thought of taking notes in the midst of a brain-splitting headache. Or they may worry that the visual disturbances and confusion that accompany their headaches will make keeping a clear and accurate record difficult. The best strategy for success is to log headaches in your diary as soon as your head pain resolves or subsides to what you feel is a manageable level. If lingering mental fogginess is making it difficult to put your thoughts on paper, keep a small audio recorder on hand and take spoken notes—you can transfer them to your diary later. Remember not to wait too long to document your headache to avoid forgetting any important details.

Alert

Don't use your diary to attempt to self-diagnose your headaches. Sometimes a severe vascular headache that seems like a migraine can be a sign of a medical emergency. Always seek the help of a qualified medical professional who specializes in headache disorders to properly diagnose and treat your head pain.

What a Headache Diary Can't Do

Remember that your headache diary is only one tool in diagnosing and treating migraine. Your doctor will take a health history from you, will perform a physical and neurological examination, and may use written or verbal screening tests and assessments to supplement your diary. He may also order lab tests and radiological exams such as CT or MRI scans.

A headache diary is also not very helpful if you aren't consistent in your entries. Try not to skip days, and remember to include the basic information outlined in the "What You Should Track" section that follows. The more thorough you are in taking notes, the more useful your diary will be to you and your health care provider.

Giving It Enough Time

The headache trends that are so valuable in the diagnosis and treatment of headache disorders won't necessarily appear in a week or two. For some people with infrequent headache, it may take several months worth of diary data for useful patterns to become clear. Be patient with the process.

What You Should Track

It's important to track not just your headaches, but also the events and circumstances that surround them. You should also note any other physical or mental symptoms you experience, even if they don't seem to be related to your headache. Things like excessive fatigue may turn out to be an early warning sign of an impending migraine. Think of your headache diary as a health and lifestyle journal, and note all food, sleep, exercise, activities, and emotional situations (such as unusual stress).

You should also note when headache episodes prevent you from participating in everyday activities, such as work, school, family time, social outings, household chores, and other responsibilities. When a headache strikes, many migraineurs withdraw into a dark, quiet, and comfortable place for recovery. And even the fear of developing a migraine may prevent you from taking part in activities you enjoy, such as going to the beach, or from planning trips. All of these things have a negative impact on your quality of life. Your doctor will use this information to help determine a course of therapy that fits your lifestyle, such as preventative migraine drugs.

Your Headache History

If you're just getting started, it's worthwhile to take some time to think about the progression of your headaches before now. If you haven't yet seen your doctor about your head pain, these details will be useful when your doctor interviews you about your medical history. This is especially true if you tend to feel anxious or pressured for time when visiting your health care provider. So gathering this information now in an unhurried and relaxed atmosphere will ensure that you have all the details your doctor needs to assist in making a diagnosis.

Some questions to consider are:

- When do you first remember the headaches starting?
- How frequent are your headaches and how long do they last?
- Is there any noticeable pattern to the timing and frequency of your headaches?
- Where is the head pain located?
- How would you describe it (e.g., throbbing, pulsating, knifelike)?
- Do you have any other symptoms along with the headache?
- Are there any signs that a headache is coming before it arrives?
- Do you notice changes in your vision before the headache begins?
- Are your headaches always the same?
- If you're a woman, do you tend to get headaches at certain points in your menstrual cycle?

- Have you noticed if specific foods, medications, stressful situations, weather changes, changes in sleep patterns, or other factors seem to trigger a headache?
- Does your headache get worse with physical activity?
- What do you do to relieve the headache, and does it work?

If you're unable to keep a headache diary prior to your appointment, or only have several days or weeks worth of diary data, it's particularly important to spend some time thinking about and answering these questions.

Diary Basics

At the least, your headache diary should track the date and time of your headache (and when it stopped), the location and nature of the head pain, any other symptoms that occurred with or before the headache, and what you were doing when the first signs of headache began. It's also useful to include food eaten, any exercise, and a notation of the weather, as bright light and temperature change can be migraine triggers.

For women, indicating your menstrual cycle on your headache diary or calendar is important. You should do this even when you don't experience headache during that time of the month. You may discover that the hormonal changes that take place during premenstruation or ovulation are associated with your headache.

 Question

I keep losing track of my headache diary. Any advice?
One sure-fire way to remember to document your headaches is to keep your diary inside a "migraine relief kit." Get a waterproof plastic box or bag and stock it with all of your migraine medications, your headache diary, compresses, an eye mask, and any other items you find helpful during migraine, such as peppermint tea for nausea.

If you've already received a diagnosis of migraine or another primary headache disorder, tracking your headaches with a diary is a key part of fine-tuning your treatment plan and uncovering any new headache triggers. In addition to tracking your headaches, you should note medication and any other treatment measures (such as retiring to a darkened room), when they took effect, and how successful they were in relieving migraine pain.

Sometimes signs of a migraine attack can appear as early as twenty-four hours prior to the actual headache, so documenting not just headache days but every day can be particularly helpful in uncovering trends. Things to note daily include any physical and emotional symptoms (even if they don't seem to be headache related); medication; beverages (including caffeine and alcohol); meals and snacks; sleep; sex; exercise; changes in weather; and home, social, and work-related activities.

Making It Easy

The simplest way to keep a headache diary is to note any headache episodes and the circumstances that surrounded them on your calendar or in your date book. If you already keep a calendar for work and family obligations, using it to log headache information too has the added benefit of providing an environmental context to migraine attacks. You may notice headaches occurring regularly alongside high-pressure meetings at work, after a strenuous aerobic class, or following family outings to the beach.

The drawback to the calendar method is that without a specific checklist of information to include in front of you, you may forget to note some essential details that could be associated with the headache, such as food, changes in temperature, or treatment notes.

One easy mnemonic, or memory device, to remember headache details is the five Ws (and one H) of journalism—who, what, where, why, when, and how. Like an investigative reporter, you're seeking out the facts that will help you determine what causes your headaches, what helps them, and when they're likely to happen again.

Rule number one is to always start with the "how":

- **How** did it start, and **how** did you treat it? Did the headache come on gradually and was it accompanied by other symptoms? What did you do to relieve the migraine pain? Was it effective?
- **Who** were you with when it occurred? Of course people aren't a migraine trigger, but who you're spending time with when a headache hits may be a clue to its cause. For example, if they happen when you're in a weekly staff meeting with your high-pressure boss, stress may be a trigger. If they only occur when you visit your cologne-loving neighbor, the odor may be causing headache.
- **What** were you doing? This question will also help you identify any headache triggers. Were you eating a particular food, exercising, sunbathing, finishing up a project on deadline, or pumping gas? Don't limit your notes to the moment the head pain starts. Jot down your main activities over the prior twenty-four hours.
- **Where** were you? Another trigger-related question. Were you in a smoke-filled bar, under the bright fluorescent lights in your office, or waking up after a late night party?
- **When** did it start and **when** did it stop? Certain types of headache, such as cluster headaches, tend to follow a time pattern. Others are related to sleep pattern disruption and menstrual cycle. The length of the headache is also an important clue.
- **Why** did it occur? Here's where you take your best guess as to what you think precipitated the migraine using the information available. You may not always know the answer to why, but as you gather diary information on your headaches over time, the patterns that determine "why" will become clearer.

Electronic and Other Options

If you feel more comfortable with a more structured way of tracking your headaches, there are many spreadsheets and printed diaries available from organizations such as the National Headache Foundation. There are software programs available for keeping headache diaries, and if you like gadgets, a PDA or wireless smart phone that you always carry with you can also be used to log headache information. You can also find online, Web-based services that provide diaries (see Appendix A for a list of resources).

Your doctor may have a specific headache diary form that he'd like you to work with. If you're looking for an easy and comprehensive headache diary format, Appendix B in the back of this book contains a blank headache log that you can photocopy and carry with you.

Essential

Keep copies of a headache log at your office, in your car, and in the other locations you spend your time so that you always have access should a headache strike. You can compile multiple logs into a single diary on a weekly basis.

Identifying Patterns

Once you've tracked your headaches, some trends should start to emerge, both in the nature of your headaches and the circumstances that surround them. The length and progression of your headache may be similar in pattern. Prodromal symptoms that occur prior to a migraine headache, such as anxiety and fatigue, may become apparent and could be reliable cues that you can use to anticipate migraine episodes.

Headache Patterns

You may notice that your headaches are happening at a certain time of day, when you encounter sensory stimuli such as flashing lights, or after you have certain foods or beverages. The location and severity of the head pain may be consistent. All of these things are important clues to a proper diagnosis.

Migraines often follow these patterns:

- One-sided, pulsating pain that tends to get worse with physical exertion
- A duration from four hours to three days
- Accompanied by nausea and vomiting
- Are alleviated by rest in a dark, quiet room
- May be followed by a period of mental confusion and sensory sensitivity

Trigger Patterns

Identifying migraine triggers is one of the most important parts of evaluating your headache diary. Since a substantial part of effective migraine treatment is avoiding known triggers, pinpointing them is critical. When something occurs in your environment two or more times prior to a headache episode, it should be considered a suspected migraine trigger. Chapter 6 explores migraine triggers in depth, but the following broad trigger categories are things you should look for as you analyze your headache diary.

- **Foods**. Because most people eat a mixed meal consisting of several foods at mealtimes, foods may take a little longer to identify as triggers. Do some detective work by reading nutritional facts labels and looking for known migraine culprits (see Chapter 17 for more on food triggers).
- **Beverages**. This includes alcohol and caffeine-containing beverages. Caffeine can both cause and soothe headache depending on the amount and frequency of its use, so it's an important element to look for when evaluating your diary.
- **Sensory stimulants**. Lights, sounds, and smells are all potential triggers.

- **Lifestyle factors**. High-stress situations, changes in regular routine, disruption of normal sleep schedules, and secondhand smoke are all lifestyle factors that can lead to a migraine.

Sharing with Your Doctor

Now that you have all this information, it's time to share it. Your headache diary can supply your doctor with a wealth of information on the circumstances surrounding your headaches, information that is key to providing a correct diagnosis and recommending effective treatment.

Your doctor may suggest that you continue to maintain your headache diary after initial diagnosis and treatment. It's also useful in tracking your progress, determining if medications and lifestyle changes are helping you, and giving your doctor the information he needs to make adjustments to medications.

Be Part of the Process

If you're headed to your first appointment for evaluation of your headache, let the doctor's office know you are bringing in a headache diary that you want to review with the provider so that appropriate time is allotted. You can also request that your doctor review your diary prior to an appointment if her schedule permits so that you can spend your time together discussing the findings.

If you've noticed patterns in your headaches, share your thoughts with your doctor. But remember to go into your appointment with an open mind. Having preconceived notions about the cause of your headaches can make diagnosis more difficult if you aren't open to hearing what your doctor has to say. Remember that you can always seek out a second opinion from another physician to confirm your diagnosis and treatment plan.

Headache and Lifestyle

Living with chronic head pain has an undeniable impact on your lifestyle. Your doctor should talk to you about what your day-to-day work and home life are like and how headache interferes with these activities. One of the factors in determining appropriate treatment is making sure it fits your lifestyle. For example, if you have to spend a lot of time driving for your job, your doctor may avoid certain drugs that could impair concentration.

 Fact

Another important function of your headache diary is to help your doctor assess the impact your headache disorder is having on your quality of life. That's why it's important to note when a severe headache keeps you home from work or school or prevents you from taking part in daily activities.

In some cases, your lifestyle may be contributing to your migraines. Shift work that disrupts sleep patterns, jobs that require being around solvents or chemicals, or bartending and waitress work in a smoke-filled environment are all possible scenarios that could trigger migraines.

Essential

Make sure your doctor knows about all dietary and herbal supplements you take. Even "natural" remedies can interact with prescription drugs or lessen their efficacy. They may also be a migraine trigger for you, so it's important to note their use to uncover any association.

Assessing Effectiveness of Treatment

Your headache diary also plays a key part in guiding your treatment plan. To determine how well your migraine medications are working and to lessen any side effects that may occur, it's important to keep an accurate record of when you take these drugs, at what dosage, and how well they alleviate your migraine pain. Did they stop the pain completely or just lessen the intensity? How long did they take to start working? Did the pain relief last for the entire length of the headache? You should also note all side effects that occur.

As you keep your diary, write down *all* of your prescription and over-the-counter medications, not just your headache medications. It's possible for some drugs to lessen the effectiveness of your migraine medication, and the doctor or neurologist who is treating your migraine may not be aware of prescriptions issued by other health care providers you see.

Recognizing Side Effects

After you begin a course of treatment for your migraine, it becomes even more important to track physical and emotional well-being on a daily basis, and not just when headache strikes. Side effects from various migraine-preventative and -abortive medications and pain-relieving drugs can run the gamut from dizziness and fatigue to gastrointestinal distress and chest pain, so watch for anything out of the ordinary that you experience.

Take care to note when side effects appear in relation to when medication is taken and how much is taken (if you aren't on a fixed dosage). Sometimes, side effects lessen over time, so pay attention to how intense they are and what impact they're having on your daily routine.

Medication Overuse

Sometimes, excessive use of pain-relieving drugs or migraine-abortive medications can actually cause persistent headaches. This is known as a medication-overuse headache or rebound headache. That's why it's important to keep careful headache diary notes on all prescription and over-the-counter medication use—including the name and amount of the drug and the time you take it.

Fact

You can build up a tolerance to pain-relieving medication. If you get tension-type headaches in addition to migraines, make sure you only use your migraine medication during a migraine attack. And certain medications, like analgesics, opioids, ergotamines, and triptans, should be used in minimal doses.

Never assume your medication dosage needs to be increased without first consulting your health care provider. If your headache diary shows that you're taking increasing amounts of medication or that you are taking your medication more often, and that the frequency of your headaches has increased, this can be a sign of medication overuse.

CHAPTER 6

Avoiding Triggers

WHEN IT COMES to a migraine, an ounce of prevention is worth a pound of cure. Once you identify the things that cause your headaches—known as migraine triggers—you can dramatically reduce the frequency of your migraine episodes. Triggers can include a wide range of environmental factors, including certain foods, beverages, chemicals, medications, and even changes in altitude. While some triggers, such as weather, may be out of your control, many can be avoided with careful planning and lifestyle changes.

What Is a Trigger?

As the name implies, a migraine trigger is something that sets off a migraine attack. It may be something you encounter in your environment, such as food and drink additives, odors, or cigarettes, or a biological change in your body, such as changing levels of hormones. Triggers are very individual, and what prompts a migraine attack in one person may not have any impact on another.

Fortunately, once identified, many triggers can be avoided. Careful reading of food and beverage labels can help you bypass many dietary triggers. The same goes for checking labels on cleaning and personal care products for chemicals, perfumes, and other odor-based triggers.

Other triggers may be controllable in theory, but harder to manage. These can include changes in your sleep schedule, medications you take (e.g., asthma or hypertension drugs), and stress. Some people have a migraine when they encounter bright or flickering lights, and while you may be able to avoid these in your home and workplace, you could encounter these stimuli outside and in other public places.

Finally, there are triggers that you have little, if any control over. These include certain weather conditions, encounters with loud sounds, and air pollution. Hormonal changes in women may also fall into this category. The best way to identify migraine triggers so you can later avoid them is to keep an ongoing headache diary. (See Chapter 5 for more on this topic.)

Lifestyle Triggers

You may find that when you're undergoing a stressful period in your life, or juggling your schedule to make accommodations for work or family commitments, you experience more headaches. Migraines commonly strike when the daily tasks of taking care of yourself—such as regular sleep, exercise, meals, and relaxation—are deprioritized and routines become erratic.

Other lifestyle habits, such as smoking and drinking, can also contribute to frequent migraines. These triggers are covered in detail later in this chapter.

Sleep

According to the National Headache Foundation, over half of migraineurs cite "changes in sleep" as a trigger for migraine attacks. Not getting enough sleep is a problem for many Americans. Adults should get seven to eight hours of sleep each evening, and most children and teens require at least nine, yet over the past twenty years, the average sleep time for both adults and adolescents has steadily decreased. And migraineurs who have six hours of sleep or less report more frequent and severe headaches than those without sleep issues.

But it's not just a lack of sleep that can prompt a migraine. Too much sleep can also be a problem. So can sleep schedules that change frequently (e.g., revolving shift-work). Any change in sleep patterns, whether it be a delayed bedtime, sleeping in on a weekend, or an impromptu afternoon nap, has the potential to trigger a headache in a migraineur.

 Fact

There is a high correlation between sleep disorders such as insomnia, narcolepsy, and sleep apnea and migraine. Because sleep problems are a trigger for migraine and migraine can increase the incidence of sleep disorders, the result can be a vicious cycle for migraineurs.

Polysomnography, or overnight sleep studies, have found that migraineurs have distinctive brain wave patterns and changes in levels of neurotransmitters like serotonin during sleep. Migraines often begin during REM (rapid eye movement) sleep, the stage or cycle of sleep during which dreaming takes place. REM is the fifth stage of sleep, and the first REM cycle during sleep happens about ninety minutes into sleep. During overnight sleep, four to six additional REM cycles, each longer than the last, occur. A three-year study of 1,698 migraineurs found that over half of migraine attacks in study subjects occurred during the hours of 4 to 9 A.M.—a time period that would be dominated by the longest stretches of REM cycle sleep. See Chapter 10 for comprehensive information on sleep and migraine.

Stress
While a large percentage of migraineurs report that stress is a trigger for headache attacks, clinical research has yet to verify a link between stress and migraine. It's possible the biological changes and fluctuations in hormones caused by chronic stress make migraine sufferers more susceptible to other headache triggers.

Another reported migraine trigger is "let down" or stress relaxation response. After periods of extreme stress, crying, or anxiety, some people may experience a migraine attack. The exact physiological relationship between stress and migraine is not understood.

Meals

Eating regular meals is an important preventative measure for migraineurs. Hypoglycemia, or low blood sugar, is a potential migraine trigger, so periods of fasting may stimulate a migraine attack. Certain stress hormones released during prolonged fasting may also contribute to migraine. If you must fast for a religious observance or medical test, break the fast with a light meal and be careful to avoid foods that may be triggers for you.

Alert

If aspartame is a migraine trigger for you, avoid Maxalt-MLT (rizatriptan benzoate) orally dissolving tablets for migraine. These contain aspartame, and there have been case reports of migraines made worse by the medication in people with aspartame sensitivity. Maxalt is also available in a standard tablet form, which contains no aspartame.

Food Triggers

Many foods and food additives have been identified as potential migraine triggers. In most cases, trigger foods contain chemicals that produce changes in body function that are believed to set the migraine attack in motion. Some commonly reported food triggers include:

- Cheese
- Chocolate
- Alcohol
- Citrus fruits
- Yeast-risen bread and bakery products
- The artificial sweetener aspartame

The Amines

Amines are derived from amino acids, and include tyramine, histamine, and beta-phenylethylamine. They are vasoactive substances (i.e., they impact the dilation and/or constriction of the blood vessels), but there may be more to the migraine/amine relationship than just blood flow, and researchers aren't sure exactly why amines seem to trigger migraine in some people.

The amines associated with migraine include:

- **Tyramine**. Many foods that are aged, such as hard cheeses and fermented or pickled foods, contain tyramine, an amino acid formed by the breakdown of proteins. So do smoked meats, chocolate, soy sauce, onions, and nuts.
- **Phenylethylamine**. This vasoconstrictor is found in chocolate.
- **Histamine**. Eggplant, spinach, and certain species of fish contain histamines naturally. Histamines are also found in foods and drinks that ferment, such as vinegars, wine and beer, and sauerkraut.

Essential

Dark chocolate is a triple trigger threat, containing caffeine, tyramine, and phenylethylamine, a vasoconstrictor. Milk chocolate contains only small amounts of tyramine, and it may be a better choice if you need a chocolate fix but are sensitive to this substance.

Tyramine, phenylethylamine, and histamine levels in food can increase as food ages, so if these are migraine triggers for you, take care to buy fish and meat fresh, store properly, and cook it in a timely manner. Don't keep leftovers around longer than a day.

Additives and Preservatives

Many food additives, colors, and preservatives are migraine triggers. These include, but are not limited to, monosodium glutamate (in large amounts), sodium nitrite, and the food dye FD&C yellow #5.

- **Monosodium glutamate (MSG).** Although probably most well known as an additive in Chinese food, MSG is found in seasonings, sauces, Parmesan cheese, and meat tenderizers.
- **Sodium nitrite.** Sodium nitrite is a preservative found in many meat products such as sausage, hot dogs, deli meat, and canned and prepackaged meat. It's also found in smoked and dehydrated meat products.
- **FD&C yellow #5 (tartrazine).** This color additive is used in many medicines, cosmetics, soft drinks, candy, and ice cream. Don't assume that a food is free of yellow #5 just because it isn't yellow; this additive is also used to create green, orange, and other colors.

Checking food labels is the best way to determine if a product contains an additive that is a trigger for you.

Beverages

Alcohol is a central nervous system depressant. It has a direct impact on brain function and can elicit migraine in some people. Many alcoholic beverages also contain histamines and high levels of tyramine, including red wine, sherry, beer, and champagne.

Many nonalcoholic beverages contain caffeine, which, unlike alcohol, stimulates the nervous system. While small amounts of caffeine can actually help ease migraine pain, in large doses caffeine becomes a dietary migraine trigger. Most people realize that caffeine is found in coffee, tea, and soft drinks, but be aware of hidden caffeine sources such as energy drinks, vitamin waters, coffee-flavored foods (e.g., ice cream and yogurt), and orange soda. Caffeine withdrawal is also a potential trigger, so keeping your caffeine intake moderate but steady is important.

Chapter 17 contains comprehensive information on potential food triggers for migraine and how to avoid them.

Weather Triggers

Changes in temperature, humidity, barometric pressure, and weather patterns have all been named as potential migraine triggers. Some people experience more migraines during certain seasons of the year. How these changes cause headache is not completely clear.

 Fact

A 2004 study from the New England Center for Headache found that the 62 percent of migraineurs studied believed that weather was a headache trigger for them. However, when headache history was matched up to actual weather data, researchers found that only 51 percent of the patients had actual weather sensitivity.

Some tips for avoiding weather-related triggers:

- **Be shady.** Bright sunlight is a very common migraine trigger and can make an in-progress migraine worse. Keep extra pairs of polarized sunglasses in your car, home, office, and anywhere else you might need them so you always have shades handy.
- **Keep cool.** If hot days are linked to your migraine pain, make sure you keep your home and work environment comfortably cool. When you're outside, try to keep covered with a broad-brimmed hat, or stay under a beach umbrella or cabana. Keeping a personal fan or water spritzer on hand can also provide refreshment.
- **Stay dry.** A dehumidifier can keep your environment dry during damp or humid weather. If humidity is a persistent trigger

for you, consider where you live. A drier climate, like New Mexico or Arizona, may help.

- **Put a lid on it**. During the winter, cold and blustery conditions may trigger migraine in some people. When the temperature dips, always wear a hat outside and keep your ears covered.
- **Freshen up**. If you also suffer from allergies and believe poor air quality may trigger your migraines, an air ionizer may help.
- **Watch the weather**. Read or watch weather reports daily to see when possible triggers are lurking in the forecast. If you're particularly sensitive to changes in barometric pressure, investing in a barometer may be helpful.

Pressure Headaches

Many weather-related headaches seem to be linked to changes in atmospheric pressure. For some people, the approach of a storm, or of a sudden cold or warm front, can precipitate a migraine

A sudden change in altitude can also trigger migraine. As the altitude goes up, the atmospheric pressure drops, and so does the oxygen level. To compensate for the reduced oxygen level, the blood vessels in the head swell, or dilate.

 Question

Can I scuba dive if I have migraines?
If your migraines are triggered by pressure changes, factors such as increased carbon dioxide levels or cold-water immersion, common to diving, may also be your migraine triggers too. Diving may not be for you. And because diving requires mental and sensory alertness, any vision loss and/or confusion you might experience during a migraine attack could prove dangerous. Talk to your doctor before trying diving.

Seasonal Triggers

Several studies examining the seasonal patterns of migraine attacks have shown that spring is the top season for hospital admissions for migraine. Both April showers and May flowers may be at the root of this trend. The damp and erratic weather of spring coupled with pollen and allergens from the season's first blooms are triggers for many migraineurs.

Summer has its own set of challenges for people living with migraine. Bright sunlight and hot weather may trigger attacks. And as days grow longer, sleep patterns are often disrupted. In fact, research on women who have migraine with aura and live in arctic regions has shown that headache attacks peak in the summer, when sunlight persists into the night, and tend to wane in the dark season (winter). Researchers hypothesized that the finding may be related to the fact that migraineurs were more likely to experience insomnia in the light season.

 Alert

Dehydration is a trigger for migraine, so always keep plenty of fluids on hand during the hot summer months. But don't go overboard on either alcohol or caffeine, as too much of either can trigger a headache. Stick to water and other nonalcoholic, decaffeinated beverages.

Fall and winter also do a number on our regular routines and sleep schedule as daylight hours shorten. And heading back-to-school and into the holiday season can bring added stress—another trigger—into your life. In fact, one Italian study of migraine in children found that attacks happened most frequently during school sessions in the fall and winter months and were least likely to occur in July.

Travel Triggers

Trips upset our daily routines, and as you're probably learning, when routines change, migraine frequently follows. When traveling, both the timing and content of meals becomes erratic. You may face temperature extremes and weather you're unaccustomed to. Sleep becomes a secondary consideration, especially during leisure travel when there's no reason to impose a strict schedule. And if you're traveling internationally or across time zones domestically, it may be days before your body and mind shake the jet lag and get back on schedule.

And of course, there's often stress involved with travel. Business travel may mean high-pressure meetings and tight schedules. Leisure trips aren't always carefree either. Even if your luggage doesn't get lost and things are moving smoothly, staying on itinerary, keeping within your budget, and coexisting with your travel companions can compound into a stress migraine trigger.

Safe Flying

If you're flying to your destination, the changes in cabin pressure that occur during takeoff and landing may be a problem. While you can't control this facet of flying, you can minimize additional triggers. Stay well hydrated, and steer clear of classic airplane food like roasted nuts or prepackaged snacks because of the high probability of preservatives and additives.

There appears to be a link between motion sickness and migraine, and people with migraine are more likely to get motion sick than those without. This is especially true in children; 45 percent of children with migraine have motion sickness, while just 5 percent of children without migraine experience motion sickness. So it's not surprising that motion sickness, from plane, train, boat, or over-the-road travel, can trigger a migraine in some people.

Avoiding Motion Sickness

All forms of transportation carry some risk for motion sickness, and consequently, migraine. There are steps you can take to stay centered and keep your stomach calm.

Passengers in a train, bus, or RV should always face forward toward the direction of travel. On an automobile trip, sitting in the front seat and looking out the window may also lessen your risk of motion sickness. Drivers are the least likely to experience motion sickness because they are focusing on the road and the motion outside and can anticipate any changes in acceleration. If you're along for the ride, try to abstain from reading or playing handheld video games, as this can precipitate motion sickness.

 Fact

Motion sickness happens when sensory input clashes. If your eyes are focusing on a near fixed object, but the balance center in your inner ear is experiencing the effects of high-speed travel, this dissonance can cause an upset stomach. This is why reading a book in the car is such a common cause of motion sickness.

Reserve a window seat when traveling by air, preferably in the front of the plane where noise levels are lower. For those migraineurs going on a cruise, try to book lower-level cabins toward the center of the boat, as these tend to experience the least amount of motion. Stay on deck when you can, as having a view of the horizon will help your body acclimate to the motion of the boat.

There are preventative treatments for motion sickness, such as scopolamine patches (Transderm-Scop) and the drug meclizine (Bonine, Dramamine). These drugs should be taken prior to travel and according to doctor's orders. Acupressure bands, worn on the wrist, may also be helpful in relieving travel-related nausea.

Sensory Triggers

Disruptive sensory input seems to trigger migraine in many people. Anything that confuses or stresses our sense of sight, sound, or smell has the potential to bring on the neurological changes that are the start of a migraine attack. While taste or touch triggers do not seem to be common, both taste and touch sensation can be altered during the course of a migraine. Also, environmental factors that involve these senses, such as the foods you eat and temperature changes you encounter, are migraine triggers. This leaves open the possibility that taste and touch centers in the brain may somehow be involved in how migraine attacks develop.

Sight

Migraineurs have an increased sensitivity to bright or flickering lights, certain colors, and pattern glare. Pattern glare is visual stress caused by a hypersensitivity to repetitive patterns, such as a checkerboard. High contrast (e.g., black and white) patterns are often associated with pattern glare. All of these visual events can be triggers for headache, and they also can worsen the intensity of a migraine attack. This sensitivity to visual stimuli is called photophobia.

Fluorescent and incandescent lighting can be too bright, and fluorescent lighting (which includes those energy-saving compact fluorescent bulbs) also generates a high-frequency flicker some migraineurs are susceptible to. Try low-wattage bulbs labeled "soft light," and don't leave bulbs exposed to the eye. A heavier light shade or opaque or dark light fixture filter may also be helpful for migraine avoidance in some people.

Screen flicker or excessive glare from a computer monitor can also precipitate a migraine attack. Try adjusting your color and contrast settings to reduce glare. Some computers allow alteration of the monitor screen frequency to minimize flicker; talk to a computer professional about making these changes.

Sound

Loud and/or persistent noise may also bring about migraine attacks in some people. Some people have a particular sensitivity to high-decibel or high-frequency sounds. This sensitivity to sound, or phonophobia, continues through a migraine attack, which is why many migraineurs seek quiet places to recover.

Smell

Whether it's a result of chemicals found in fumes or a reaction to scent, exposure to certain odors can cause migraine in some people. This sensitivity to odors can range from traditionally "pleasant" but strong smells like perfumes and scented candles, to fumes from chemicals, secondhand smoke, pollution, and automobile exhaust. A 2004 study of Atlanta-based migraineurs found that smell was a migraine trigger in close to half of study subjects. Pungent odors are the most likely to become migraine triggers.

Drug and Chemical Triggers

While there are many useful medications available for the treatment of migraines, there are also an abundance of prescription medications, over-the-counter remedies, and illegal drugs that affect the brain and vascular system and act as potential migraine triggers. Perhaps the most common among adults is alcohol, a central nervous system depressant, covered earlier in this chapter.

With an estimated 45 million adult American smokers, cigarettes are also one of the more common migraine triggers. Cigarette smoke—both firsthand and secondhand—may trigger a migraine attack, and the full health effects of the over 4,000 chemicals found in cigarette smoke are not fully understood.

 Fact

Illegal or recreational drugs can also be migraine triggers. Cocaine use may be of particular concern. Addicts seeking drug rehabilitation treatment who have a history of migraine should be closely supervised, as withdrawal also causes an increase in migraine attacks.

Aside from increasing the frequency of migraines and the risk of heart disease and lung cancer, studies have shown that smoking increases risk of stroke sevenfold in women who have migraine with aura. If you smoke and have migraines, talk to your doctor about a plan for quitting. Nicotine replacement therapies such as patches and gum can be a useful aid for smoking cessation. However, their use should be carefully supervised, as sudden withdrawal from nicotine can also be a migraine trigger.

Prescription and OTC Medications

Because prescription and over-the-counter medications must undergo extensive clinical trials and scientific scrutiny before they are approved for market, including full disclosure on all statistically significant side effects, they are perhaps the most well-studied triggers. The following drugs have been associated with migraine attacks:

- Hypertension drugs
- Nitroglycerin
- Erectile dysfunction drugs: Sildenafil (Viagra), vardenafil (Levitra), and tadalafil (Cialis)
- Anti-asthma medications
- Estrogens

Hormonal Triggers

Up to 70 percent of women with migraine name hormonal changes related to their menstrual cycle as a major migraine trigger. Research has established a fairly clear link between the hormone estrogen and migraine frequency in female migraineurs. Estrogen effects on the brain are complex but can include changes in the levels of the neurotransmitter serotonin, which is linked to the brain changes that occur in migraine.

When estrogen is rising or is holding steady, most female migraineurs experience fewer menstrual-related migraines. It is not uncommon for the frequency of migraine to decrease in pregnancy when estrogen levels are rising rapidly. Alternately, sudden drops in estrogen levels can precipitate migraine. Women who take birth control pills with high levels of estrogen as a contraceptive or to regulate their cycle are also at higher risk for migraine, especially with those preparations where the pill taken during the last seven days of a twenty-eight day cycle is actually an inactive substance. This withdrawal is the trigger for menstruation but leaves the woman most vulnerable to a migraine attack during that week. Migraines tend to resurface during the postpartum period, as estrogen levels drop, but there is some evidence that breastfeeding will extend the migraine improvement period for many women.

 Fact

Before menarche, or first menstruation, girls experience migraine at roughly the same rate as boys, and some research shows the boys may even slightly outnumber the girls. But after puberty hits, female migraineurs outnumber males two to one, and by adulthood, the spread widens to three to one.

While these are the most common observations, the effects of estrogen on migraine are likely quite complex and often unpredictable. For example, estrogen-based hormone replacement therapy (HRT) used for relief of menopausal symptoms may be a migraine trigger for some women. Of great concern for older women who are smokers and who have experienced migraine with aura, there may be a small increase in the risk of stroke when taking birth control or hormone replacement therapy.

Menstrual Migraine

Migraine that is directly related to the menstrual cycle with no other identifiable triggers is called menstrual migraine. Most women who have menstrual-related migraines do not consistently experience aura. Fortunately, women who can link their migraines to a predictable menstrual calendar typically have an advantage in treating and preventing their attacks. Using migraine preventative treatments immediately before, during, and again immediately after menstruation is highly effective in many women.

Menopause and Beyond

For women with migraines linked to their menstrual cycle, menopause often brings about a decrease in migraine frequency. However, for women who have surgical menopause (i.e., menopause brought about by surgical removal of both ovaries, or caused by ovarian failure following hysterectomy), migraines may actually worsen.

Part of this likely relates to the abrupt drop in hormone levels immediately following surgery, but over time the increase is likely associated with the higher rate of estrogen replacement therapy (ERT) or hormone replacement therapy (HRT) in women who have undergone surgical menopause. In postmenopausal women with a history of migraine who require ERT or HRT, continuous transdermal (i.e., through the skin) treatment that provides a low and steady amount of estrogen to the body is preferred to keep hormone fluctuations to a minimum. This may be in the form of a skin patch or gel. See Chapter 11 for more information on migraine and hormones.

CHAPTER 7

Acute Treatment Options

MIGRAINE TREATMENT FALLS into two categories—acute or preventative (also called prophylactic). Acute treatment is an analgesic, or pain-relieving, medication or therapy that is taken when a migraine begins. It is designed to stop or alleviate the pain and other symptoms of a migraine attack. When acute treatment fails to stop head pain, then a more potent rescue medication is required. It's important not to overuse either acute or rescue migraine medications, as overuse can cause more frequent, or "rebound" headaches.

Pain Relievers (Nonopioid)

Nonopioid analgesics are pain relievers that do not contain opioid, or narcotic, drugs. These drugs are recommended by the U.S. Headache Consortium as the first line of treatment for people with mild-to-moderate pain and disability from migraine. Nonsteroidal anti-inflammatory drugs (NSAIDs) are effective because they reduce inflammation and ease mild head pain. Aspirin, ibuprofen (Advil, Motrin), naproxen (Aleve), and ketorolac (Toradol) are all NSAID drugs. Acetaminophen is not an NSAID, but it is a nonopioid analgesic.

Caffeine is sometimes combined with nonopioid analgesics to relieve migraine pain, and in combination can boost the potency of these drugs by approximately 40 percent. Excedrin Migraine is a combination acetaminophen, aspirin, and caffeine formula. In addition, nonopioid analgesics are often combined with antiemetics, or antinausea, medication to reduce vomiting and stomach upset in migraine.

L., Essential

Liquid gel capsules or caplets, such as Advil Migraine, may be a better choice for fast head pain relief than standard tablets because the medication is predissolved and therefore is absorbed more quickly in the body.

Side Effects of NSAIDs

Because they are not addictive, nonopioid analgesics are frequently a first treatment choice for migraine headache. These medications should be used with caution, as they can have significant side effects. These include fluid retention (edema), nausea, vomiting, diarrhea, constipation, reduced appetite, heartburn, and fatigue. People with kidney problems, liver problems, asthma, heart disease, and ulcers should consult their doctor before taking NSAIDs for migraine, as these drugs can make these conditions worse. If you take NSAIDs, you should not drink alcohol, as this can increase your chance of stomach bleeding. Some NSAIDs can increase your sensitivity to the sun, so avoid prolonged sun exposure and use sunscreen when taking them.

Side Effects of Acetaminophen

Acetaminophen is often a preferred drug for mild migraine pain because it has virtually no side effects. However, if taken in large doses, acetaminophen can cause liver damage, so caution should be taken to stay within the recommended dosage. Many prescription and over-the-counter drugs, including some cough and cold remedies, contain acetaminophen—so always check with your doctor before combining other medications with acetaminophen because of the risk of accidental overdose. There are a number of drugs that interact with acetaminophen and with NSAIDs, so you should tell your doctor about all prescription and over-the-counter medications you take if he prescribes these drugs for your migraines.

Pain Relievers (Opioid)

Opioid pain relievers are narcotics, and because they can cause physical dependence and have many side effects, they are used with great caution in migraine treatment. They are only prescribed to rescue those patients who experience moderate to severe migraines, and usually only after other migraine medications have been used without success. It's important to note that there are currently no opioid drugs that are FDA-approved specifically for migraine relief. Most have general pain-relief indications, but many have been used in clinical trials and as an "off label" migraine therapy by physicians.

Opioids that may be prescribed for migraine treatment include butorphanol (Stadol), oxycodone (Oxycontin), morphine (Avinza, Kadian, MS Contin, MSIR, Oramorph, Rescudose, Roxanol), meperidine (Demerol), fentanyl (Actiq), levorphanol (Levo-Dromoran), propoxyphene (Darvon), and methadone (Diskets, Dolophine, Methadose). These drugs are available in either oral, suppository, injectable (i.e., intravenously or subcutaneously), or transdermal (i.e., skin patch) formulations. Butorphanol tartrate is available in a generic nasal spray form for faster pain relief. Codeine, the mildest opioid analgesic, is usually used in combination with acetaminophen or other nonopioid analgesics (Tylenol #3).

 Question

What is "off-label" drug use?
When a doctor prescribes a drug for a use that has not been approved by the U.S. Food and Drug Administration in the drug's official labeling, it is called "off-label" use, which may be appropriate when it is backed by published medical literature or recommended by medical organizations or other government health agencies.

To prevent drug dependence and rebound headache, opioid analgesics should be used no more frequently than two days a week. Overuse of opioids causes a patient to become physically dependent on the drug, and increasingly tolerant of doses, which have to be raised to achieve similar efficacy. When opioid use is stopped abruptly in someone who has become dependant on the drug, not only do headaches recur with increased severity but also symptoms of withdrawal can occur, including sweating, abdominal pain and nausea, vomiting, sweating, and diarrhea.

Rescue Therapy

Because of their potential for physical dependence, opioids are usually reserved as rescue, or abortive, migraine therapies. This means that they are a second-line treatment that is used only when nonopioid therapies are ineffective and migraine pain is severe. If your migraines don't respond to preventative therapies because they are infrequent and unpredictable, and they are moderately severe to severe in pain intensity, your physician may prescribe these drugs as a backup to nonopioid analgesics.

Side Effects of Opioids

Side effects associated with opioids include nausea, vomiting, forgetfulness, confusion, fatigue, constipation, and itching. They are sedatives, so should never be used before driving or operating machinery. Opioids should not be taken with alcohol, and they must be used with caution in people with reduced liver or kidney function. Because opioids depress respiration (decrease breathing rate), they are not a good treatment choice for anyone suffering from lung problems such as chronic bronchial asthma, emphysema, or chronic obstructive pulmonary disease (COPD).

Ergot Derivatives

Ergot derivatives (dihydroergotamine and ergotamine) are an older class of migraine medications. Because of the high incidence of side effects, especially nausea as an immediate side effect, complex vascular problems when used over the long term, and the availability of more effective therapies, these drugs are typically only used in patients who have severe side effects or allergies to other migraine medication. Ergot derivatives only relieve the pain symptoms of migraine, while other symptoms associated with a migraine attack may linger. Ergotamine can actually prolong aura in patients who experience migraine with aura, and the drugs can also increase nausea and vomiting.

Alert

In March 2007, the U.S. FDA sent warning letters to twenty drug companies, instructing them to stop selling unapproved medications containing ergotamine tartrate for the treatment of migraine, including several popular ergotamine and belladonna combination drugs previously marketed for migraine prevention. FDA-approved ergotamine drugs were not affected by the action.

Fast-acting formulations of ergot derivatives are available in pills that dissolve under the tongue (Ergomar), injections (DHE-45), and nasal sprays (Migranal).

Side Effects of Ergot Derivatives

Ergot derivatives can cause troublesome side effects, including nausea, abdominal cramps, dizziness, and dry mouth. Like opioids, frequent use of ergot derivatives results in increased tolerance and physical dependence on the drug. Too much of the drug can also trigger rebound or medication overuse headaches. When ergot derivatives are prescribed, they should be taken no more frequently than twice a week.

Because these drugs cause blood vessel constriction, they can also cause a condition known as peripheral vasospasm, which can restrict arterial blood flow and cause ischemia (tissue death) and potentially gangrene. Signs of this less common but potentially serious side effect include leg cramps and coldness, numbness, or pain in the hands or feet.

 Fact

Dexamethasone is a corticosteroid that is administered intravenously to treat intractable migraine (i.e., migraine lasting longer than seventy-two hours). While several published case reports note the drug's efficacy, clinical trials on the drug have found no significant benefits. Further research is needed to see if corticosteroids have a role in migraine care.

If you take triptans, you should not take ergot derivatives, as the combination can cause a serious drug interaction. And if you are a woman who is pregnant or nursing, or if you have a history of heart disease, severe high blood pressure, angina, coronary artery disease (CAD), reduced liver or kidney function, or peripheral vascular disease, you should not take ergot derivatives. People with mild high blood pressure or hyperthyroidism should consult with their doctor before taking these drugs.

Combination Formulations

Ergot derivatives are often combined with other medications to increase their efficacy and reduce side effects. Ergotamine and caffeine combinations are available in generic form and under the brand names Cafergot and Migergot. These formulations are available in pill or suppository form. Suppositories may be preferred when nausea and vomiting are severe.

Triptans

Triptans are a class of drugs known as serotonin receptor agonists. They were specifically designed as migraine therapy, and are the most commonly prescribe migraine medication today. Serotonin is a neurotransmitter, or brain chemical, that helps to regulate mood, appetite, sleep, and other brain/body functions. Triptans work by inhibiting the transmission of signals in certain nerve centers of the brainstem, and in doing so they seem to be able to terminate or reduce the complicated cascade of inflammation and vascular changes going on in the head that are associated with migraine head pain and migraine-related nausea, vomiting, and photophobia (sensitivity to light).

Alert

If you take antidepressants, talk to your doctor before taking a triptan drug. Selective serotonin reuptake inhibitors (SSRI) and selective serotonin/norepinephrine reuptake inhibitors (SNRI) are antidepressants that interact with triptans, and a life-threatening condition called serotonin syndrome can occur, though rarely, in patients taking both drugs.

The triptans include sumatriptan succinate (Imitrex), zolmitriptan (Zomig), eletriptan hydrobromide (Relpax), naratriptan hydrochloride (Amerge, Naramig), rizatriptan (Maxalt), frovatriptan succinate (Frova), and almotriptan malate (Axert). These drugs are available in various formulations, including oral drugs, nasal sprays, and injections (depending on the type of triptan). The injectable form is frequently prescribed for those migraineurs who experience severe vomiting during a migraine attack.

When to Take Triptans

Triptan drugs work best when they are taken as soon as a migraine attack begins. Taking a triptan early also reduces side effects and decreases the chance of migraine recurring in the next twenty-four hours. Studies show that on average, triptans abort up to 80 percent of migraine headaches within two hours. Triptans can sometimes be used as a preventative, or prophylactic medication, particularly in the case of menstrual migraine. Chapter 8 has more details on triptans as prophylactics.

Side Effects of Triptans

People who take an SSRI, SNRI, or monoamine oxidase (MAO) inhibitor should not take triptans without discussing risks carefully with their doctor, as these combinations can rarely cause serious and even life-threatening interactions. Triptans should also not be taken with ergot derivatives (see previous section). Triptans can also cause some mild side effects including:

- Flushing of the skin
- Tingling of the skin
- Tightness in the chest and/or throat
- Drowsiness or fatigue
- Dizziness
- Muscle weakness
- Burning at injection site (for injectable sumatriptan)

People who have a history of heart attack, stroke, angina, or atherosclerosis should not take triptans because triptans can constrict blood vessels. These drugs are not approved for use in pregnant women or in children under age eighteen, although they are sometimes prescribed for adolescents on an "off-label" basis when other treatment methods fail.

Antinausea Medications

Nausea and vomiting are common features of migraine. Approximately 80 percent of migraine attacks are accompanied by nausea, and an estimated 30 percent are accompanied by vomiting. Antiemetics are drugs that treat nausea and vomiting. They are sometimes combined with analgesics, ergotamines, or triptans (although triptans have their own nausea-relieving properties). Adding an antiemetic to migraine therapy—either within a combination drug or as a separate medication—can help you keep oral medications down and ease stomach discomfort.

Antiemetics—What's Available

Antiemetics are available in oral, injectable, suppository, and intravenous formulations. Oral formulations are most useful when they are taken early in a migraine episode, as vomiting later in an attack can prevent proper absorption. Suppositories and injections are helpful if medicine is not staying down. Intravenous formulations of prochlorperazine (Compazine) or chlorpromazine (Thorazine) may be administered in a doctor's office, urgent care, or emergency department setting.

Prescription antiemetics include ondansetron (Zofran), promethazine (Phenergan), and metoclopramide (Reglan). Metoclopramide also stimulates the gastrointestinal system, providing the added benefit of improving the absorption of other analgesics. This results in faster pain relief when the drug is taken in conjunction with an analgesic.

Side Effects of Antiemetics

Drugs with antiemetic properties fall into several different pharmaceutical categories, so their side effects can vary. Some antiemetics, including promethazine, include antihistamines that can cause dizziness, drowsiness, and dry mouth. Prochloraperazine and chlorpromazine are both antipsychotic drugs that can cause these same side effects, along with constipation, chills, blurred vision, and nasal congestion.

One particular side effect of the antipsychotic drugs used as antiemetics, called acute dystonia, is uncommon but striking when it occurs. This consists of a sustained set of movements affecting the eyes or the head and neck or the limbs that can last for hours. It is a benign phenomenon, but can be quite distressing. Fortunately it is quickly relieved by anticholinergic medications such as diphenhydramine (Benadryl).

Metoclopramide increases gastrointestinal motility, so it may cause diarrhea in some people. In rare cases, long-term use of meto-clopramide can cause tardive dyskinesia—involuntary tremors or muscle spasms that persist even after the drug is no longer used.

 Fact

The newest class of migraine drugs under development is known as oral calcitonin-gene-related peptide (CGRP) receptor antago-nists. These drugs work by blocking the CGRP neurotransmitter, a pain-related brain chemical that is elevated during a migraine attack. Trials have shown that these drugs are similar in efficacy to triptans and may have fewer side effects.

Avoiding Rebound Headaches

Overuse of some acute migraine medications can result in more fre-quent, and sometimes more intense, headache episodes. This phe-nomenon is known as a rebound, or medication overuse, headache. Rebound headaches may turn into a chronic daily headache that is similar in nature to a tension-type headache, or they may be migraine headaches that occur with increased frequency.

All classes of acute migraine medications have the potential to cause rebound headache when used more than two or three times a week. Unfortunately, this perpetuates a vicious cycle—you take more medication to treat the ensuing headache.

Recognizing a Rebound Headache

It can be difficult to recognize a headache caused by medication overuse, particularly if you have always experienced frequent migraine attacks. Although any new patterns or symptoms of head pain should be evaluated by your health care provider, the following signs may be a red flag that you are experiencing rebound headaches:

- Your headaches have increased in frequency to daily or almost daily.
- You are taking more headache medication more frequently, and it's less effective in relieving your head pain.
- Your headaches have changed in nature or severity (e.g., your head pain is a constant dull ache instead of a throb; your head pain is occurring in different places).
- Your head pain returns several hours after taking a dose of medication.

Treating a Rebound Headache

Once a rebound headache develops, the best way to treat it is to stop taking the medication that triggered it. Your doctor may recommend that you taper off the medication, or use a different drug type. Always consult with your health care provider before stopping a drug abruptly. It can take anywhere from a week to several months to completely break the rebound cycle, and your head pain may worsen before it improves. If you have become dependant on an opioid pain reliever, you may experience uncomfortable withdrawal symptoms. In some cases, your health care provider may recommend supervised drug withdrawal in a hospital setting. In most cases of simple nonopioid analgesic overuse, you can handle rebound treatment on your own with rest, relaxation, and cold compresses.

Bed Rest, Compresses, and Cold Packs

There are many, simple nonpharmaceutical treatments that you can begin at home at the first sign of an impending migraine. While they won't stop migraine pain completely, they can provide some relief while you wait for medication to take effect and can ease the discomfort of any breakthrough pain. They also have the benefit of being inexpensive and side-effect-free.

Rest is the simplest and most common of these pain-relief measures. An estimated 58 percent of all migraine attacks experienced by migraineurs between the ages of twenty and sixty-four result in some bed rest, and women spend an average of six hours in bed due to migraine compared to four and a half hours for men. The American Migraine Study found that roughly one-third of all migraineurs require bed rest during a migraine attack.

Bed Rest

Retreating to a dark, restful place when head pain begins is almost instinctual for many migraineurs. Since a migraine causes light and sound sensitivity and is relieved by sleep, it makes sense to unplug the phone, dim the lights, and crawl under the covers until the attack passes. If you have odor sensitivities, banish any scented candles or air fresheners from the area.

Lying down provides some minor relief from the throbbing vascular headache of migraine, which is made worse by physical activity. If at all possible, try and withdraw from the outside stresses of work and other responsibilities. Read Chapter 10 for more important information on creating a restful migraine recovery environment.

Compresses and Cold Packs

Most migraineurs find that cold compresses, or packs, are more effective than heat packs in easing head pain. Although there is no published research on the topic, this may be because cold reduces inflammation. There are many cold packs on the market targeted specifically for migraine pain relief.

A cold pack can be as simple as a washcloth soaked in cold water. Cold compresses filled with gel material hug the face closely, retain cold, and may be more comfortable than an ice pack on sensitive skin. There are also commercially available cold gel patches that adhere to the forehead and can be useful in soothing migraine head pain.

Biofeedback

Biofeedback is a nondrug therapy that has been extensively studied and proven effective in clinical trials to relieve migraine head pain, and in some cases, to prevent the occurrence of migraine. As the name implies, biofeedback is a system of monitoring your body's biological signals, such as temperature, heart rate, and muscle tension, and learning how to regulate those functions through relaxation and visualization techniques. It requires formal training with a health psychologist, headache specialist, or physical therapist. These health care providers often have special certification in biofeedback training.

Essential

Both The Association for Applied Psychophysiology and Biofeedback (AAPB) and the Biofeedback Certification Institute of America (BCIA) can provide references to certified biofeedback therapists in your area. Visit the AAPB Web site at www.aapb.org and the BCIA Web site at www.bcia.org.

When biofeedback is effective, it also gives you a sense of control and empowerment over your head pain, which provides an additional psychological benefit to dealing with migraine. It is also used prophylactically, along with relaxation techniques, to prevent migraine episodes in some patients.

Biofeedback is an ideal treatment option for children because it avoids the side effects of most migraine drugs, many of which have not been tested extensively in younger populations. And because, with regular practice, it is a lifelong skill, it may be more cost-effective than medication over time.

The Mind-Body Connection

The idea of controlling autonomic, or involuntary, bodily functions like heart rate and temperature may sound a bit new age or far-fetched to some. But medical doctors and psychologists alike have long recognized the connection between emotional well-being and physical health. Many physical functions are adversely affected by stress and anxiety, so using psychological techniques to reduce stress can have a very real impact on your health.

The physical impact of stress on the body is one that most people don't often think about, but it has a tremendous impact on both migraine and overall health and well-being. When you are in a stressful situation, the blood vessels in the brain and muscles dilate, or expand, and the heart rate and blood pressure rise increase your oxygen supply. Blood vessels near the skin and in your hands and feet dilate, or contract. All these physiological responses are designed to protect the body in circumstances of real danger—known as the fight or flight syndrome. For example, reduced blood flow near the skin means that you will bleed less if cut, and increased oxygen supply helps you to defend yourself or flee a dangerous situation. This biological programming has helped promote human survival for thousands of years.

The problem with the stress response is that in today's world, you rarely need to fight off the kind of life-or-death dangers we are physiologically programmed to deal with. Instead, regular everyday annoyances, such as traffic jams or too much to do at work can lead to what becomes habitual stress. Your body can become chronically "stuck" in a stress response state, which can contribute to major health problems—including headache and migraine.

Biofeedback Training

Biofeedback training can take anywhere from several weeks to several months to complete, depending on the frequency of the sessions and the training program. If you decide to try out biofeedback, you must commit to regular at-home practice of the techniques taught in training. This is critical to internalizing biofeedback skills and giving yourself the best tools available to treat and prevent migraine episodes. Your biofeedback therapist may provide you with special audiotapes or CDs and/or a home temperature sensor to help aid you in these sessions. She may also ask you to log temperature readings before and after you practice.

Fact

Some migraineurs who master biofeedback techniques may still require medications occasionally, but the frequency of need and the dosage is often reduced. But even if you find that you need a combination of therapies to effectively manage your migraines, biofeedback is still a useful skill for long-term health and well-being.

Training usually begins with an introduction to the equipment involved. Thermal sensors are attached to the fingers. Cold fingers indicate tension and restricted peripheral blood flow. Electromyogram (EMG) sensors or electrodes are placed on the body to measure muscle tension. A visual display and/or audible representation of these signals provides the "feedback," which a patient is taught to read and interpret. The feedback may be displayed on a computer screen, or it may be in the form of flashing lights, a numerical display, a paper readout, or a pattern of sounds.

Your biofeedback trainer will then introduce you to some basic relaxation, visualization, and breathing techniques. The breathing exercises typically involve deep breathing from the diaphragm. For relaxation and visualization exercises, your provider will put you in a comfortable seated or reclining position in a quiet space. The lights may be dimmed and temperature adjusted to make the environment more comfortable. Relaxation exercises, sometimes called progressive relaxation, teach an awareness of muscle tension and relaxation by focusing on tightening, and then relaxing, one muscle group at a time. Visualization exercises involve clearing your mind and picturing yourself in a safe, peaceful, and warm place where you are free of stress, relaxed, and comfortable. Your provider will serve as coach, talking you through these exercises.

A baseline finger temperature and EMG reading is taken before relaxation and breathing exercises. Once you are hooked up to the equipment, you can see what state of relaxation your body is in and monitor changes as you practice relaxation, breathing, and visualization. A rise in hand temperature indicates that you are increasing the blood flow in your hands (your peripheral circulation). This may be the mechanism that helps to reduce or prevent migraine head pain by diverting excess blood flow from the brain. Muscle tension can also contribute to or exacerbate head pain, so learning to relax muscles through biofeedback can also be helpful in migraine treatment.

 Fact

Some studies have indicated that neurofeedback, which is biofeedback that uses an EEG to measure brain waves via sensors placed on the head, may be useful in identifying and perhaps preventing the cortical spreading depression associated with the onset of a migraine attack.

Biofeedback ultimately teaches you how to end that habitual stress response and relax mentally and physically. When the feedback monitors tell you that you have increased your hand temperature or reduced your muscle tension, you have tangible evidence that the technique is effective. That feedback may also serve as a psychological "reward," which can make relaxation more emotionally fulfilling and easier to attain over time.

CHAPTER 8

Prophylactic Medications

IF YOUR MIGRAINES are frequent, significantly impact your daily life, or your acute medications just aren't working well enough for you, your doctor may prescribe a prophylactic, or preventative, medication. As of early 2008, the FDA had approved four drugs for migraine prophylaxis—topiramate (Topamax), divalproex sodium (Depakote), propranolol (Inderal), and timolol (Blocadren). Classes of drugs that have demonstrated promise as migraine preventatives include antiepileptics (AEDs), antidepressants, beta-blockers, calcium channel antagonists, and NSAIDs. It's important to note that prophylactic migraine medications may not eliminate your need for acute medications completely.

Antiepileptic Drugs (AEDs)

Antiepileptic drugs, sometimes called antiseizure or anticonvulsant drugs, are a class of medications used in the treatment of epilepsy and other brain-based disorders. They are thought to prevent migraines by increasing levels of the neurotransmitter GABA, which helps to suppress the spreading cortical depression (abnormal electrical activity in the visual cortex of the brain) that triggers a migraine attack. In clinical studies, several AEDs have demonstrated an ability to reduce both the frequency and intensity of migraine attacks.

While there are a number of AEDs prescribed as migraine preventatives, only divalproex sodium valproate (Depakote) and topiramate (Topamax) have been approved for this use by the U.S. Food and Drug Administration. Other AEDs that are not FDA approved but are sometimes prescribed "off-label" for the prevention of migraine include gabepentin (Neurontin), carbamazepine (Tegretol), phenytoin (Dilantin), and lamotrigine (Lamictal).

Alert

If you suffer from hemiplegic migraines, a severe but rare type of migraine with aura that causes weakness or paralysis on one side of the body and can result in coma, your doctor will recommend prophylactic medication. Calcium channel blockers are effective prophylaxis. Chapter 1 has more information on hemiplegic migraine.

If you and your doctor decide that one of the AED drugs are a good choice for you, you will be started on a low dose that is gradually titrated, or increased, in order to minimize side effects and find the optimal dosage level. This may occur over a period of weeks or even months. When starting on an AED, it's important to maintain your headache diary carefully so you can gauge how effective the treatment is and document what side effects, if any, you are experiencing.

Side Effects of AEDs

Fatigue, paresthesia (tingling of the hands and/or feet), and dizziness are common side effects of Topamax. So are gastrointestinal issues such as nausea and diarrhea, and related weight loss. Other less common side effects include depression, anxiety, insomnia, vision problems, and difficulty concentrating.

A rare but serious side effect of Topamax is a condition known as metabolic acidosis, where bicarbonate levels in the blood become elevated. Symptoms include hyperventilation, irregular heartbeat, fatigue, loss of appetite, and mental confusion.

Side effects of Depakote may include hair loss, nausea and vomiting, weight gain, weakness, dizziness, tremor, and sleepiness. Depakote is a central nervous system (CNS) depressant, so it should not be taken with other CNS depressants, including alcohol. Increased levels of ammonia in the blood can occur in some people taking Depakote, which can cause lethargy, vomiting, and a change in mental status. The drug may also cause thrombocytopenia, or a low blood platelet count. Periodic blood tests may be required to monitor for these conditions in patients taking Depakote.

Some side effects of AED drugs can mask the presence of other health conditions. Always tell your doctor about any side effects you experience in conjunction with your migraine medication, whether you're just starting out on the drug or have been taking it for some time.

Who Should Not Take AEDs

If you have existing kidney or liver problems, AED drugs may not be an appropriate treatment choice for your migraines. People with urea cycle disorders should not take Depakote because of the risk of hyperammonemic encephalopathy, excessive levels of ammonia in the bloodstream that lead to swelling of the brain. Depending on the drug you are prescribed, you may have to undergo regular blood tests to ensure that your liver function and/or blood values remain healthy.

AEDs should not be used during pregnancy if at all possible. For example, Depakote ingestion during pregnancy has been associated with neural tube and other birth defects.

If you already take prescription drugs, supplements, or over-the-counter medications for migraines or to treat other health conditions, make sure your doctor is aware. AEDs may interact with these substances, causing serious side effects or affecting the potency of one or more drugs. For example, barbiturates, or combination analgesics containing barbiturates, can interact with valproate and potentially cause serious neurological complications.

Antidepressants

Clinical studies have found several antidepressants to be useful in migraine prevention. They are thought to prevent migraines by regulating the levels of serotonin, norepinephrine, and other neurotransmitters in the brain.

Amitriptyline (Elavil, Endep) is an antidepressant and antianxiety medication that was also one of the earliest and most-studied migraine prophylactics. Amitriptyline is a tricyclic antidepressant, an older class of antidepressant drugs. Other tricyclics have been studied for migraine prevention, but amitriptyline is the only one that has been proven effective in controlled clinical trials. It is considered a first-line drug in migraine prophylaxis.

The other, newer, antidepressant drug that has shown some efficacy in migraine prevention is fluoxetine, or Prozac. Fluoxetine is a selective serotonin reuptake inhibitor drug, so should be used with caution, if at all, in people who are taking triptans because of the risk of serotonin syndrome.

Side Effects of Antidepressants

Tricyclic antidepressants cause a number of troublesome side effects, including dry mouth, dizziness, nausea, constipation, weight gain, anxiety, photosensitivity (i.e., sensitivity to sunlight), and fatigue. Orthostatic hypotension, a sudden drop in blood pressure when changing position, may also occur. Less common but potentially more serious side effects can include loss of libido, blurred vision, high blood pressure, and increased heart rate. If taken in too high of a dose, TCAs can cause seizures, stroke, or heart attack.

Fluoxetine can also cause nausea, weight gain, anxiety, insomnia, and fatigue, although these side effects often lessen or disappear over time. In some people, the drug may more rarely cause skin rashes, increased blood pressure, seizures, and vasculitis.

Antidepressants should never be abruptly stopped (i.e., "cold turkey") because doing so can cause dizziness, headache, muscle aches, nausea, and anxiety.

Who Should Not Take Antidepressants

If you take an MAO inhibitor, you should not take TCAs or fluoxetine because of the risk of a life-threatening drug interaction. Any MAO inhibitor must be stopped two weeks prior to starting these antidepressants.

Essential

The antidepressant drug classes serotonin reuptake inhibitors (SSRIs) and selective serotonin/norepinephrine reuptake inhibitors (SNRIs) can cause serotonin syndrome when taking in conjunction with triptan drugs. Symptoms of serotonin syndrome include irregular heartbeat, increased body temperature, hallucinations, and fluctuating blood pressure.

Antidepressants should be prescribed with care and monitored closely in patients with liver, kidney, or heart disease. Certain antidepressants are not recommended for use in people who are recovering from myocardial infarction (heart attack).

Beta-Blockers

Beta-blockers are drugs that relax blood vessels and block the effects of adrenaline in the body. Traditionally used to treat heart disease, beta-blockers became recognized for their usefulness in the prevention of migraine in the 1970s. Those that are FDA approved for this use include propranolol hydrochloride (Inderal) and timolol maleate (Blocadren). Other beta-blockers that have been studied in migraine prevention and may be prescribed "off label" for the purpose, but are not FDA approved for this use include atenolol (Tenormin), nadolol (Corgard), and metoprolol (Lopressor, Toprol).

Propranolol is the oldest and most widely studied of the migraine prophylactic beta-blockers to date. It is also the least expensive of the first-line migraine preventative drugs (in its generic form).

Side Effects of Beta-Blockers

Potential side effects of beta-blockers include fatigue, sleep problems, depression, decreased physical endurance, and impotence. Propranolol and other beta-blockers decrease blood pressure and could cause dizziness and fainting in people with normal to low blood pressure as a result.

 Fact

The FDA has not yet approved any medication for the prevention of migraine in children and teenagers. However, the Cochrane Review, an evidence-based review of available research on health care interventions, found that the beta-blocker propranolol hydrochloride and the calcium channel blocker flunarizine (available in Canada only) may be effective prophylactics for this age group.

Who Should Not Take Beta-Blockers

Migraineurs who have lung or breathing problems such as asthma and chronic obstructive pulmonary disease (COPD) should not take beta-blockers, as these drugs can cause breathing to deteriorate. They are also not recommended for use in people who have bradycardia (slow heart rate) or electrical conduction problems with their heart. Beta-blockers can interact with or impact the efficacy of a number of over-the-counter and prescription medications; make sure your doctor is aware of all the drugs you take to prevent dangerous interactions.

Calcium Channel Blockers

Like beta-blockers, calcium channel blockers are a class of medications traditionally used to treat cardiovascular conditions such as hypertension and irregular heart rhythms. They block the absorption of calcium into the heart muscle and vascular system, "relaxing" the cardiovascular system and increasing blood flow to the heart. They are also thought to regulate serotonin levels, which may explain their efficacy in migraine prevention.

Some studies have shown that verapamil (Calan) and nifedipine (Procardia) may be useful in the prevention of migraine. Other calcium channel blockers, such as nimodipine, have demonstrated conflicting results. None of these drugs are FDA approved for use in migraine prevention.

Fact

Taken orally, the calcium channel blocker verapamil has shown promise in preventing hemiplegic migraine in several clinical studies. Case studies suggest that intravenous infusion of the drug may help to abort hemiplegic migraines already in progress.

Side Effects of Calcium Channel Blockers

Potential side effects of calcium channel blockers include constipation, edema (swelling), and low blood pressure causing dizziness or even fainting.

If you are prescribed a calcium channel blocker, you should not take it with grapefruit or grapefruit juice because these decrease the efficacy of the drug. Alcohol should also be avoided, as it can magnify some side effects and interfere with the activity of the drug.

Who Should Not Take Calcium Channel Blockers

People with certain preexisting health conditions should use calcium channel blockers under a doctor's recommendation and close supervision. Because there are more effective migraine prophylactics available, your doctor may recommend that you avoid calcium channel blockers completely if you have very low blood pressure, heart failure, or impaired liver or kidney function.

Pregnant women should avoid the use of calcium channel blockers because of the risk of birth defects.

Nonsteroidal Anti-Inflammatory Drugs (NSAIDs)

Nonsteroidal anti-inflammatory drugs (or NSAIDs) are considered a second-line preventative treatment for migraine. They are often recommended when preexisting health conditions make first-line treatments inadvisable, or when first-line treatments just aren't effective. They may also be useful to those who can't tolerate the side effects of antiepileptics, beta-blockers, and antidepressants.

For women who suffer from menstrual migraine, NSAID drugs are highly effective. The drugs are usually started about seven days prior to the start of the menstrual period and taken two to three times daily, depending on the drug and dosage.

Essential

Triptan drugs aren't typically used for the prevention of migraine—except in the case of menstrual migraine, where triptans have shown some efficacy as migraine prophylactics. Published studies of naratriptan (Amerge) and frovatriptan (Frova) show the drugs can prevent menstrual migraine in many women.

NSAIDs used for migraine prevention include aspirin (or acetylsalicylic acid), naproxen sodium (Aleve), and ibuprofen (Advil). Although many NSAIDs are sold as over-the-counter drugs, you should work with your health care provider to determine what kind and dosage of the medication is best for your particular situation.

Side Effects of NSAIDs

Some NSAIDs can increase your sensitivity to the sun, so avoid prolonged sun exposure and use sunscreen when taking them. Other side effects associated with NSAIDs include fluid retention (edema), nausea, vomiting, diarrhea, heartburn, and fatigue.

Taking NSAIDs with alcohol can increase your chance of stomach bleeding and should be avoided. If you take lithium, methotrexate, or any diuretics, NSAIDS can impact the therapeutic action of these drugs. Check with your doctor about the possible interaction of NSAIDs with other medications or supplements you are taking.

Who Should Not Take NSAIDs

If you have stomach ulcers, asthma, heart disease, or kidney or liver problems, certain NSAIDs can aggravate these conditions. Anyone with an allergy to aspirin or to an NSAID should not take these drugs. Aspirin itself or nonaspirin salicylates should never be used in children or teenagers who have flu-like or viral symptoms because it can increase the risk of developing Reyes Syndrome, a rare but potentially fatal disease that can cause serious damage to the liver, brain, and other organ systems.

Because NSAIDs inhibit platelet function (decrease the ability of the blood to clot), they should be avoided in people who take other blood-thinning drugs (anticoagulants) or who are scheduled for surgery.

Angiotensin Blockade Agents

In addition to the beta-blockers and calcium channel blockers, a third type of heart drug, angiotensin blockade agents, has also shown great potential in migraine prevention. These drugs include certain angiotensin-converting enzyme (ACE) inhibitors, angiotensin receptor blockers (ARBs), and a subtype of ARBs known as angiotensin II receptor antagonists.

Angiotensin blockage agents work to balance fluid and electrolyte levels in the blood and are approved and prescribed for use in treating high blood pressure. As such, they may be a good treatment choice for migraineurs who also suffer from hypertension or prehypertension. It's not yet fully understood exactly how these medications work to prevent migraine, but researchers have theorized that it may be related to their ability to block the action of angiotensin II, a chemical that constricts blood vessels.

Fact

> A 2002 metanalysis published in the American Journal of Medicine found that among the 12,110 patients studied, the risk of headache was one-third lower in those patients taking an angiotensin II receptor antagonist than in those who did not.

In the early 2000s, two separate Norwegian studies found that the ACE inhibitor lisinopril (Zestril) and the ARB candesartan (Atacand) cut total days with migraine by more than half in study subjects. Other studies of the drugs have reached similar conclusions.

The angiotensin II receptor antagonist, olmesartan (Benicar), also showed very promising results in a 2006 U.S. study, with subjects reporting an 82.5 percent reduction in the frequency of their migraines and a 45 percent reduction in migraine severity.

Side Effects of Angiotensin Blockade Agents

Angiotensin blockade agents seem to have fewer severe side effects than some of the other prophylactic drugs for migraine. Commonly reported side effects are lightheadedness or dizziness, low blood pressure, fatigue, increased blood potassium levels, and a metallic or salty taste in the mouth.

Who Should Not Take Angiotensin Blockade Agents

Most people with impaired kidney function or liver disease should avoid angiotensin blockade agents, as should anyone with a known allergy to drugs in this class. Because of their ability to increase potassium levels in the bloodstream, these drugs should not be taken with potassium supplements or foods or medicines that are known to increase potassium (including potassium-fortified salt substitutes). They should also not be used with diuretics.

Some angiotensin blockade agents can increase side effects of the drug lithium, and anyone taking both of these medications should be closely monitored by his physician. These drugs may also interact with other medications; again, always speak with your doctor about possible interactions with your current prescription and supplement regimen.

Other Migraine Preventatives

Researchers continue to investigate new ways to prevent migraine, with some surprising results. Sometimes, medications and therapies that were thought to be effective only in easing the pain of an active migraine attack have proven themselves useful as migraine prophylactics. And other treatments have been discovered quite by accident from completely different fields of medicine.

Botulinum Toxin

Most people recognize Botox as a cosmetic surgical agent injected to reduce or eliminate fine lines and wrinkles in the skin (known clinically as "hyperfunctional facial lines"), though it has several other indications for the treatment of complex neurological and medical disorders. In the 1990s, when the drug was initially being studied as a cosmetic therapy, researchers noticed a decrease in the frequency and severity of migraine headache in some study subjects who were given Botox. This prompted further investigation into the use of the drug as a migraine treatment, and there are now dozens of published studies on the topic.

Botulinum toxin type A (BoNTA; Botox), is a neurotoxin that is cultured from the anaerobic bacterium Clostridium botulinum, an organism found in soil and water. Once cultured, the toxin is sterilized and vacuum-dried. It is mixed with saline and injected with a fine needle just under the skin, usually into the forehead. The toxin causes short-term muscle paralysis in the area it is injected into, and may have some impact on the nerve fibers that could explain its usefulness in short-term migraine prevention.

As of early 2008, Botox was not yet approved by the FDA for the treatment of chronic migraine, and Allergan (the manufacturer of Botox) was completing phase III clinical trials of the drug for this use.

Botox has few side effects when administered in proper doses by a health care professional. The area surrounding the injection site can become weak if the toxin spreads. Although this is the desired therapeutic effect of the drug, it can be a problem if it spreads to the eyes (causing drooping), throat (causing difficulty swallowing), or other unintended areas.

Question

Will one series of Botox injections stop my migraines forever?
No known migraine prophylactic agent is 100 percent effective. And the effects of botulinum toxin on nerves and muscles are temporary, lasting four to six months before another treatment is necessary. Remember that Botox is not yet FDA approved for migraine prevention, so any use of the drug for this purpose is considered "experimental."

Double-Duty Drugs

Several of the analgesic drugs used for acute migraine pain are also sometimes prescribed, with varying success, for migraine prevention. The nonsteroidal anti-inflammatory drugs have already been covered in depth earlier in this chapter.

An older analgesic drug class that has some benefit in migraine prevention is that of the ergot derivatives. One such drug, methysergide (Sansert), is an oral tablet approved for use as a migraine prophylactic. Though it is not effective in treating migraines once they have begun, it is particularly effective as a prophylactic. Unfortunately, because of its side effects, some potentially quite serious with long-term consequences for kidney and cardiovascular function, methysergide is typically not a front-line choice for migraine prevention. See Chapter 7 for more details on ergot derivatives.

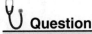 **Question**

> **Will any supplements help prevent migraines?**
> Feverfew (Tanacetum parthenium), magnesium, coenzyme Q10, and vitamin B2 (riboflavin) have all shown initial promise in clinical trials as migraine prophylactics. Chapter 9 covers these complementary therapies in more detail.

Biofeedback, Take Two

Biofeedback—the practice of self-monitoring your body's biological signals and learning how to regulate them through relaxation and visualization techniques—is a proven therapy in the treatment of migraine head pain. It has also been studied as a migraine preventative. The effectiveness of the therapy may be due to the ability of biofeedback and relaxation therapy to reduce stress, a known trigger of migraines.

Because of the psychological benefits and lack of side effects of biofeedback therapy, it is an ideal treatment choice for children and pregnant women, for whom the risks of drug therapy are either too great, or unknown. Turn to Chapter 7 to find out more information on biofeedback therapy.

CHAPTER 9

Alternative and Complementary Medicine

"ALTERNATIVE" MEDICINE ISN'T so alternative anymore, with billions of dollars spent on supplements, acupuncture, and other untraditional therapies by American consumers each year. Alternative medicine, perhaps more accurately defined here as complementary medicine, is the practice of typically noninvasive, natural therapies and techniques used to complement, or enhance, traditional Western medicine. There are many promising therapies for migraine treatment and prevention that are outside of the medical mainstream, but there is also just as much junk science. Be an informed consumer, know what the science says, and work with your health care provider to select complementary therapies that count.

Vitamin B₂ (Riboflavin)

Most vitamins, minerals, and dietary supplements are relatively inexpensive when compared to prescription migraine drugs. And because they have been around considerably longer than most drugs, many have proven safety and low-side-effect profiles. This makes them a good alternative for migraineurs, especially those who can't tolerate the side effects of prescription migraine drugs.

Clinical studies of vitamin B_2 or riboflavin, as a migraine treatment have pointed toward the efficacy of the vitamin in migraine prevention. Riboflavin seems to have little effect on the length of a migraine attack, but it can reduce the severity of a migraine attack and appears to have a significant impact on reducing migraine frequency in most studies. One trial found that doses of 400 mg daily for three months reduced migraine days by half. But yet another study indicated that a dose as low as 25 mg may have similar efficacy.

 Fact

> Riboflavin combined with beta-blockers (e.g., metoprolol, biso-prolol) may be an effective migraine prophylaxis. A study published in the journal Headache found that both treatments have similar levels of efficacy but work through different physiological mechanisms, and combining the two may result in better migraine prevention.

Further large-scale, long-term studies are needed to confirm the value of riboflavin therapy as a migraine prophylactic. But researchers seem to agree that riboflavin is best used as an adjunct, or companion, therapy to other migraine treatments. It is largely safe, inexpensive, and apparently effective with few side effects.

How It Works

Riboflavin helps to regulate cellular metabolism and increase energy production in the mitochondria of the cells. It has been theorized that migraineurs may have reduced energy activity within the mitochondria of the cerebral blood vessels, and this could be why riboflavin works as a migraine therapy.

Dietary sources of riboflavin include milk and dairy products, eggs, cereals, meats, and dark green vegetables. Riboflavin is light sensitive, and the riboflavin content of these foods quickly degrades with prolonged exposure to light (e.g., milk in a cardboard container may retain riboflavin better than milk in a glass bottle). Riboflavin deficiency is uncommon, and is usually a result of a diet that is inadequate in these riboflavin-rich foods. However, it can also be caused by certain gastrointestinal disorders and liver disease. And the condition rarely occurs on its own; it is usually in connection with other B-vitamin deficiencies.

Side Effects and Cautions

Side effects of riboflavin supplementation include upset stomach, diarrhea, and flavinuria—or dark yellow urine. Flavinuria is a harmless side effect. Some people may experience an allergic reaction to riboflavin supplementation, indicated by a skin rash, breathing problems, or swelling.

Riboflavin can interfere with the efficacy of certain antibiotics and sulfa drugs, so tell your doctor if you are prescribed these medications while taking riboflavin supplementation—you may have to suspend your supplements temporarily.

Niacin

Niacin, also known as nicotinic acid or vitamin B$_3$, has been used intravenously and orally as both a preventative and an abortive treatment for migraine. There have been case reports suggesting niacin's effectiveness published in the medical literature, as well as a handful of small studies. Whether the usefulness of the drug was related to the action of the drug itself or to a placebo effect is unclear. Unfortunately, as of early 2008 there were not yet any well-designed, randomized, controlled trials of niacin as a migraine treatment.

 Fact

A 2007 Belgian study found that thioctic acid (also known as alpha-lipoic acid) may be helpful in preventing the frequency of migraine attacks after three months of therapy. Further studies are needed to confirm whether or not this natural antioxidant is safe and effective over the long term.

How It Works

Researchers believe niacin may be effective in stopping a migraine because of its vasodilatory action (it opens blood vessels). This vasodilatory action may also cause side effects such as flushing of the skin, a warm sensation in the face or neck, and fainting or dizziness. Other reported side effects of niacin include itching, dry skin, and nausea. Many of these side effects appear when niacin therapy is first started or when dosage is increased, and then gradually decrease over time.

Magnesium

Unlike niacin, magnesium does have a few well-controlled, randomized trials indicating its efficacy in migraine prevention. One study of oral magnesium oxide supplementation found that a dose of 600 mg daily over twelve weeks significantly decreased the frequency of migraine attacks. Other small but well-designed studies have found that magnesium supplementation may also be a safe and effective prophylactic therapy for children, and for women suffering from menstrual migraine.

Intravenous magnesium sulfate has shown promise as an acute therapy for migraines in progress. One small 2001 study found that the treatment eliminated head pain in 86 percent of the patients studied. Another study of emergency room treatment in migraineurs found that intravenous administration of magnesium sulfate was just as effective in reducing migraine head pain as IV infusion of metoclopramide.

How It Works

How does magnesium work? The mineral helps to regulate serotonin and other neurotransmitter function, and promotes muscle relaxation, among other things.

Research suggests that migraineurs have lower levels of magnesium in the body than most people, which could explain the mineral's effectiveness in migraine treatment.

Essential

The best way to get essential vitamins and minerals is through a varied and healthy diet. The vitamins and minerals found in your food are better absorbed than supplements, taste better, and are cheaper in the long run.

A deficiency of magnesium can actually cause headache and sensitivity to light, which could explain its effectiveness in migraine treatment. Magnesium deficiency is not a common condition and occurs most often in people who have a malabsorption problem (problems absorbing nutrients from food), in chronic alcoholics, and as a side effect of certain medications. People with a calcium deficiency may also have a related magnesium deficiency.

Side Effects and Cautions

Poor nutrition also has the ability to affect magnesium levels in the body. High sugar, fat, and phosphate intake through processed foods can affect the absorption of magnesium. Red meat, green leafy vegetables, and whole grain cereals are all good dietary sources of magnesium.

 Alert

Some foods rich in magnesium may also be a trigger for migraine in some people. Almonds, cashews, soybeans, and seafood are all abundant sources of magnesium, but have been reported to trigger attacks in some migraineurs.

Oral magnesium supplements can cause gastrointestinal distress at high doses—including nausea, bloating, and diarrhea. When taken as a supplement at levels high above recommended dosage, magnesium can be toxic to the body. Symptoms of a magnesium supplement overdose include erratic heartbeat, skin flushing, dizziness, confusion, muscle weakness, and loss of consciousness. Excess magnesium taken in dietary form does not cause side effects because the body excretes it naturally.

Coenzyme Q10

Coenzyme Q10 (CoQ10) is a substance that is found naturally throughout the body and has also been synthesized in a supplement form. It is an antioxidant that plays a role in energy production of the cells, and the highest levels of CoQ10 can be found in the organ systems that consume the most energy (e.g., the heart, brain, liver, and kidneys). Levels of coenzyme Q10 decrease with age and with the presence of some chronic health conditions, such as cancer, heart disease, diabetes, and others.

In supplement form, coenzyme Q10 appears to have some effectiveness as a migraine preventative. It is usually taken in a water-soluble formulation (e.g., a liquid gel capsule), and is prescribed in daily doses, sometimes divided (i.e., taken at intervals throughout the day).

 Fact

A study of children and adolescent migraineurs published in 2007 found a CoQ10 deficiency in study subjects. When daily supplementation of CoQ10 was prescribed, migraine frequency and disability were both reduced.

Unfortunately, there are only a handful of studies on CoQ10 to date, and most are small or not scientifically rigorous. While larger, long-term trials of CoQ10 are needed, it is worth noting that studies to date have found that CoQ10 supplementation cut migraine headache days by more than half in some patients.

Side Effects and Cautions

There are few side effects associated with CoQ10, and those that have been reported are typically mild. These include mild nausea, light sensitivity, fatigue, and dizziness. Potential allergic reactions to the supplement include rash and itching. Most side effects resolve quickly without treatment.

CoQ10 can decrease blood pressure and blood glucose levels, so people with pre-existing hypotension (low blood pressure) and hypoglycemia (low blood sugar) should only use the supplement with caution under a doctor's care. The supplement may interact with some prescription and over-the-counter drugs, so always consult your doctor and/or pharmacist when adding it to your medication regimen.

Herbal Supplements

While herbal preparations have been used for thousands of years to treat everything from headache to the plague, the advent of formal clinical study on these herbs is relatively recent. As a result, the body of modern scientific literature—in the form of large, controlled, randomized, and long-term trials—is small on most herbal supplements in comparison to the body of literature on commercial prescription and over-the-counter drugs. This is attributable to several factors, including the large amount of research funding provided by pharmaceutical companies, and the differences in regulatory processes between drugs and supplements.

Several herbal supplements have been studied for use in migraine treatment, and the research data, though limited, provides some indication of their efficacy. Those herbs that have the most positive research results in relation to migraine treatment are described below.

Feverfew

Feverfew (*Tanacetum parthenium, Chrysanthemum parthenium*) is a medicinal herb that has been used to treat various ailments—

including headache—for centuries. The feverfew bush, which is also known commonly as bachelor's buttons, is a fast-growing plant that has daisylike flowers when in bloom. The herb is native to Europe but is now widespread throughout North and South America.

Essential

The Federal Trade Commission (FTC) and the FDA are two good sources of information about disreputable supplement distributors and known health care scams. You can visit them online at www.ftc.gov and www.fda.gov.

While feverfew leaves are sometimes taken medicinally, commercial preparations of the supplement may contain leaves, flowers, and stems processed into capsule, tablet, or liquid extract formulations. Due to variations in plant varieties and manufacturing processes, the strength and quality of feverfew supplements you may find at your local health food store can fluctuate widely (see the Smart Supplementation section that follows).

Studies of feverfew in migraine treatment have had mixed results. The herb may have some benefit as a preventative medication, but as is the case with most supplements for migraine prevention, there have not been enough large-scale, long-term, controlled trials to reach a definitive conclusion on the herb. In addition, several of the existing studies test not feverfew alone but in combination with another substance.

For example, a sublingual (under the tongue) compound of feverfew and ginger was used in one small study to treat head pain at the beginning of a migraine attack, and close to half of the subjects reported no pain two hours after treatment. And another study combined feverfew with the herb white willow (*Salix alba*) to produce a compound that reduced the frequency, severity, and duration of migraine after three months of daily supplementation.

But some research has determined that feverfew is not any more effective than placebo in managing migraine pain. Clearly, further research is necessary to determine whether feverfew holds promise as a migraine treatment. In the meantime, it may be an option for those who cannot tolerate the side effects of other prescription and over-the-counter medications.

Feverfew has a few potential but uncommon side effects, including nausea, bloating, canker sores, irritation of the lips and tongue, and changes in sense of taste. Sudden withdrawal of the herb after long-term use has also been associated with sleeplessness, headache, anxiety, and muscle pain.

 Alert

If you have an existing allergy to plants in the daisy family, including ragweed, you may be allergic to feverfew. Signs of an allergic reaction include rash, itching, and swelling. In severe cases, an allergic reaction can slow or even stop breathing due to swelling of the airway.

Butterbur

Butterbur (*Petasites hybridus*), also know as butterfly dock, bog rhubarb, and blatterdock, has been used for medicinal purposes since the fourteenth century. This perennial plant is small with large, rhubarblike leaves and spiky flowers, and has a large rhizome, or root, which is used in herbal preparations.

While butterbur has been studied extensively as a treatment for allergies because of its anti-inflammatory and antihistamine properties, less research exists on its role as a migraine treatment. Most studies involve an extract of the butterbur root taken in tablet form, known commercially as Petadolex. While further long-term, well-designed studies of the herb are needed, existing studies indicate that butterbur has some efficacy as a migraine preventative.

Like feverfew, butterbur is related to ragweed and can cause an allergic reaction in anyone with an existing ragweed allergy. The herb has not been studied extensively enough to document all potential side effects, but those that have been reported in conjunction with clinical trials include nausea, belching, and other mild digestive complaints.

Question

Is butterbur a safe alternative for children?
A 2005 German study of over 100 children and adolescents studied the effectiveness and safety of butterbur in migraine treatment. Researchers found that daily supplementation with butterbur extract over a period of four months cut the frequency of migraine attacks in half for 77 percent of patients. Adverse events (i.e., side effects) were also low.

Smart Supplementation

When you go to the store to buy a bottle of aspirin, there may be many brands on the shelf, but you can be assured that all are of a similar quality and strength (as indicated on the package). Dietary supplements, and especially herbal supplements, are a different story. The way an herb is grown, the parts of the plant used, the manner in which it is harvested and stored, and the processing and manufacturing methods used all play a part in the quality and strength of the supplement that ends up in your local store.

Like prescription and over-the-counter drugs, dietary supplements are regulated by the U.S. Food and Drug Administration (FDA). But unlike drugs, supplements do not have to undergo any approval process before reaching the consumer market. As such, the quality of supplement products can vary widely.

Look for the designations "U.S.P." (U.S. Pharmacopeia) or "NF" (National Formulary) on the label when selecting supplements.

These indicate that the supplement manufacturer observes quality control and good manufacturing practices and that the product meets nationally recognized strength, quality, purity, packaging, and labeling standards as recommended by the FDA.

 Fact

Legislation known as the Dietary Supplement Health and Education Act (DSHEA) was passed in 1994 in an effort to standardize the manufacture, labeling, composition, and safety of botanicals and supplements. The FDA is expected to fully implement these regulations by the year 2010.

Acupuncture

Acupuncture is a common treatment in traditional Chinese medicine (TCM) that has gained momentum in Western medicine. The therapy involves the placement of thin, disposable needles just under the skin, which are targeted to locations on the body known as "acupoints." The goal of acupuncture is to harmonize the energy flow within the body.

How It Works

The insertion of acupuncture needles stimulates an increase in pain-killing endorphins and serotonin levels in the blood and brain. Acupoints for migraine treatment will vary by patient and symptoms but include locations on the ears, face, forehead, neck, hand, or forearm.

In 2007, a randomized and controlled trial of acupuncture coupled with the migraine drug rizatriptan found that the acupuncture group had better outcomes than the group who took rizatriptan alone. And an earlier trial that coupled acupuncture with flunarizine had similar findings.

Another study of 300 migraineurs who underwent twelve sessions of acupuncture over a three-month period found that the therapy resulted in twenty-two fewer headache days per year, 15 percent less medication use, 25 percent fewer visits to the doctor, and 15 percent fewer sick days attributed to headache compared to those who didn't have the treatments.

But not all the research on acupuncture in migraine backs its clinical efficacy. A large German trial found that what is known as "sham acupuncture," which is a type of placebo involving the superficial and nontherapeutic insertion of acupuncture needles, is just as effective as regular acupuncture treatment.

Sham acupuncture was used as a placebo treatment in the control group (the group of study participants not receiving the treatment being studied) of the trial. The control group experienced levels of migraine pain relief similar to the group who did receive genuine acupuncture, indicating that it may have been the patients' expectations for the treatment that produced the beneficial results, not the treatment itself. However, some acupuncture researchers have questioned the results of these trials, stating that even sham acupuncture stimulates nerve activity and hormonal changes involved in the relief of pain.

Cost and Safety

When performed by an experienced licensed acupuncturist, acupuncture is extremely safe. The needles used are disposable and the skin is swabbed with disinfectant prior to puncture, so the risk of infection is very slim. Needles are inserted just under the skin, so bleeding is minimal, if it occurs at all. The only side effect may be a slight burning sensation at the site of the needle entry.

Not all health insurance plans will cover acupuncture treatments, which can make it an expensive treatment option for some. However, given that studies have documented a significant decrease in both the amount of prescription medication and sick days from work among migraineurs who undergo the treatment, it may be even more cost-effective than traditional medical options for some.

Avoiding Quackery

Because the world of supplements and nontraditional medicine is more loosely regulated than mainstream medicine, there is more opportunity for consumer fraud and subpar or ineffective treatments.

The best way to get quality treatment is to find a quality, credentialed practitioner. Get to know the national professional groups and credentialing organizations for the type of practitioner you wish to see. You can also check with your local and state departments of health to ensure that an alternative practitioner is licensed to practice what he or she claims, and to check for any consumer complaints.

Alternative Practitioners

Health care providers that practice alternative or complementary medicine cover a broad spectrum of disciplines. They can range from "traditional" doctors like general practitioners, internists, and even neurologists who advocate the use of select complementary therapies when appropriate, to "alternative" providers like naturopaths, homeopaths, acupuncturists, and practitioners of traditional Chinese medicine who specialize in these therapies.

 Fact

The designation OMD stands for Oriental Medicine Doctor, and signifies a health care provider who specializes in the practice of traditional Chinese medicine (or TCM). An OMD has undergone a doctorate-level degree program in TCM at an accredited university.

Board certification in a specific discipline is the best way to verify that a health care provider has the knowledge and experience to administer a particular therapy. Typically, most health care board certifications require many hours of training and study, followed by a rigorous examination.

Several medical organizations exist for the board certification of acupuncturists. These include the National Certification Commission for Acupuncture and Oriental Medicine (NCCAOM), American Board of Medical Acupuncture (ABMA), and the American Manual Medicine Association (AMMA). If a doctor or health care practitioner is board certified by one of these organizations, he will have these credentials:

- Diplomate in Acupuncture (NCCAOM)
- Diplomate of the American Board of Medical Acupuncture; or DABMA (ABMA)
- National Board Certified Practical Acupuncturist; or P.Ac., and the National Board Diplomate Acupuncturist, or Dipl.Ac. (AMMA)

In addition, practitioners are often certified at the state level. For example, in New York, you must be a licensed doctor or dentist and meet acupuncture education and training requirements to qualify for certification. Check with the health department or department of consumer affairs in your state to find out what the criteria is in your area.

A naturopathic physician (ND or NMD), is a doctor who specializes in natural medicine. Naturopaths avoid drugs and surgery and instead use a variety of complementary therapies, including herbs, acupuncture, bodywork, aromatherapy, and homeopathy. They also practice more "traditional" areas of care such as nutrition therapy and counseling. Preventative medicine is one emphasis of naturopathy, as is treating the "whole person," or holistic health care.

Alert

Not all naturopathic physicians are licensed or board certified acupuncturists. If you are seeking acupuncture from an ND, be sure to inquire about his or her credentials in the treatment first. Similarly, medical doctors (MDs) must also have licensing and/or board certification in acupuncture to administer the treatment.

The American Naturopathic Certification Board (ANCB) is the organization that board certifies practitioners in naturopathic medicine. The designation CTN (Certified Traditional Naturopath) indicates a naturopathic physician has received this certification. Many states also regulate the licensing of naturopaths; check with the department of health to find out the policy in your area.

What to Watch Out For

Perhaps you aren't seeing a complementary practitioner, but are interested in trying out a supplement, vitamin, or other alternative migraine treatment. Of course, it's always best to check with your primary care physician before trying any new treatment—even one touted as "natural"—since the medication you may already be taking can interact with even natural treatments. But there are some signs that the treatment you are considering may be a scam.

- **If it sounds too good to be true, it probably is.** Pills, powders, and juices that tout themselves as "miracle cures" should raise a big red flag. A cure is something we just don't have for migraine disease yet.
- **Watch out for he said/she said.** Advertisements that are full of testimonials from "satisfied customers" and even doctors, but that lack hard clinical information and studies, are probably not backed by any scientific proof of efficacy.
- **Beware of one-size-fits-all claims.** If a product purports to treat everything from dandruff to diabetes, it is probably a scam. While some supplements and vitamins can be beneficial for multiple conditions, a laundry list of treatable diseases is a sign of a hoax.

Complementary therapies can be a wonderful addition to your migraine treatment regimen. With some basic consumer shopping smarts, a little research, and the guidance of your health care provider, you can use these "natural" treatments to your best advantage.

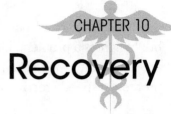

CHAPTER 10

Recovery

MEDICATION IS ONLY one part of treating a migraine attack. Feeling physically and emotionally better after a migraine attack takes time, and even with migraine medication that works for you, the effects of migraine can linger for days. Many migraineurs experience a postdromal phase—a period of time following a migraine headache where fatigue, mental cloudiness, and mild head pain are common. Giving yourself time to recover in a healthy and comfortable environment is important.

A Safe Space

Migraines attack all the senses, causing pain; nausea; and sensitivity to light, sound, odors, and in some cases, touch. So it's critical to have a comfortable, dim, quiet, and fragrance-free space in your home that you can retreat to whenever a migraine hits. The bedroom is a logical choice—there's a comfortable place to lie down and you mentally associate the room with rest. However, any room of your home will do as long as it's properly prepared.

Think about your specific migraine symptoms and what supplies you should have on hand to best combat them. Keep your migraine prescriptions and OTC drugs at bedside if possible (if you have children, make sure all medication is safely secured in childproof containers). If nausea and vomiting is a persistent problem, a pan or other receptacle is a necessity. Water and mints (if tolerated) can help clean out your mouth if you feel too ill to get out of bed. If sound intensifies your head pain, earplugs may be helpful. If sensitivity to bright light is a problem, have a soft eye mask at your bedside. There are also many ways to adjust the design of your space in order to promote a speedy recovery.

Migraine-Friendly Design

If your bedroom gets lots of sunlight, it's important that you be able to block light effectively at a moment's notice. Blackout shades or curtain liners can help darken your room, and they have the added benefit of being good noise insulators. If you find that you're most comfortable with some low ambient light, install a dimmer switch or a lamp that has dimming capabilities.

Essential

While you may enjoy scented home and personal products and candles, the odors often aggravate the pain and nausea of migraine. Designating your bedroom or other recovery space a fragrance-free zone will prevent any odor sensitivities that pop up during a migraine attack.

Making your recovery space quiet may be your biggest challenge. Make sure your phone has a ringer that can be turned off. If your bedroom is in a high-traffic area of your home, consider converting a remote room of your house into a recovery space. If circumstances make complete quiet hard to achieve, a white-noise machine can help block out unwanted sound. There are also sound machines available that play ocean surf, rain, and other natural environmental sounds at a low level, which may help you relax while blocking out ambient noise.

Other Environmental Considerations

Comfortable temperature and humidity levels can also play a role in recovery. Depending on weather patterns and air quality in the part of the country you live in, you may occasionally need some extra help above and beyond central heating and/or air conditioning units. Store an extra fan, dehumidifier, and/or air filtration unit in the closet to have on hand as needed. The more comfortable you are, the easier it is to rest and speed your recovery.

 Fact

Several studies that include self-reported treatment techniques of migraineurs indicate that applying cold compresses to the head is one of the most commonly used pain-relief techniques. Cold application may help ease pain by reducing inflammation.

Comfort Measures

Some migraineurs experience increased sensitivity to touch, so a set of high-thread-count sheets, soft blankets, and comfortable lounge-wear or pajamas can make a world of difference. You may find that elevating your head helps to alleviate lingering head pain, so have extra pillows on hand to adjust as needed. Nonpharmaceutical pain relief in the form of cool compresses, massage, and relaxation techniques is also an important part of recovery for many migraineurs. They also have the added benefits of minimal cost and no side effects. There is limited research on the effectiveness of massage in migraine treatment and recovery. Studies surveying migraine patients show that applying manual pressure to the pain points on the head is a frequently used method of alleviating head pain. Chapter 7 has more information on the use of compresses and relaxation techniques for migraine treatment, and Chapter 9 explores the use of other body-work techniques.

Sleep

The healing powers of sleep for headache pain have been recognized in medical literature for over a century. In the late 1800s, researchers noted how sleep relieved headache, and physicians frequently prescribed hypnotic sedative drugs to induce sleep and treat pain.

Migraine research in the 1970s and 1980s began to explore the relationship of sleep to headache recovery. Several studies of migraineurs during this time found that those who slept during a migraine attack were able to recover more quickly than those who didn't sleep or merely dozed. The restorative power of sleep for headache resolution has also been noted by migraineurs in several large-scale surveys.

Alert

Children with migraine are more likely to suffer from sleep disturbances and associated behavioral problems than their peers without migraine. This may include insomnia and resistance to bedtime. Educating children and parents about proper sleep hygiene and reinforcing positive sleep behaviors is important to reducing migraine frequency.

More recently, large-scale studies have demonstrated that migraineurs are more likely to experience sleep disorders (e.g., insomnia, sleep apnea). Those that are sleep deprived (i.e., sleep six hours or less per night) tend to experience more severe and more frequent attacks. Researchers at the Headache Center of Atlanta conducted a study of over 1,200 migraineurs, and found that 85 percent of patients choose to sleep or rest to recover from headache, and 75 percent of patients reported that they had no choice but to sleep or rest to resolve their head pain.

The Sleep-Migraine Connection

The exact mechanisms by which sleep helps to relieve migraine are unknown. But researchers have uncovered some clues. Migraineurs who experience attacks that wake them from sleep may have increased REM-stage sleep cycles. During REM sleep, the neurotransmitter changes in the brain, including decreases in serotonin production, could be the trigger for the appearance of a migraine attack.

 Fact

Studies have shown that people who suffer from migraine are three times as likely to experience excessive daytime sleepiness. This may be due to the higher incidence of sleep disorders in migraineurs or from the sleep-robbing impact of migraine attacks and subsequent migraine-related disability.

Another biological clue to the sleep-migraine connection may be melatonin, a hormone secreted by the pineal gland. Melatonin helps to regulate sleep cycles and also has anti-inflammatory properties. Migraineurs may have lower levels of this hormone than the general population. Further large-scale studies are needed to determine whether or not melatonin supplementation is an effective treatment option for migraine patients.

Sleep in Migraine Prevention

Sleep hygiene, or the practice of getting regular, healthy amounts of sleep, can be a great preventative strategy in migraine treatment as well. A University of North Carolina study found that good sleep hygiene reduced the frequency of migraine 29 percent and the intensity of migraine pain 40 percent, compared to migraineurs who didn't practice good sleep hygiene.

Chapter 14 offers some helpful strategies for achieving healthy sleep patterns with proper sleep hygiene.

Minimizing Stress

Unfortunately, the rest of the world doesn't stop when a migraine hits, and the daily responsibilities of work, school, family, and other commitments can make recovery more of a challenge. Because rest speeds recovery for most migraineurs, the ideal situation would be to stay home and call in sick to all responsibilities for the day. However, that is frequently not an option for many people.

 Fact

Stress is a known trigger for migraine attacks and can also make an active migraine worse. A UK survey conducted by the Migraine Action Association found that 66 percent of migraineurs surveyed pointed to stress as a primary migraine trigger.

Make things easier for yourself by laying the groundwork now. Educate the people around you about your condition, have alternative arrangements made for regular commitments and responsibilities, and always have migraine supplies within an arm's reach. Advance planning can make a big difference in recovery time when migraine strikes.

Have a Plan

When calling in sick to work is not an option, try to shift your schedule an hour or two to allow time for your pain relievers to take effect. It can be very helpful to have a discussion with your supervisor about your condition on a day when you're feeling well, explaining how migraine disables you (e.g., visual problems, nausea, pain) and how her flexibility will help you to be a more productive employee. If your employer is prepared in advance and is willing to work with you, you'll feel less stressed about making the call when you need to. Chapter 14 has more information on your rights and responsibilities in the workplace.

Keep the numbers of several local cab companies handy, along with an extra stash of cash for cab fare in case you have to go to work or to an appointment during a migraine attack. Never get behind the wheel when a migraine is causing visual disturbance (aura or otherwise), when head pain or nausea will divert your full attention from the road, or when you're taking medication that alters your ability to drive.

Keep your freezer stocked with prepared, nutritious meals that require minimal time and effort to get on the table. While nausea may make food the furthest thing from your mind during a migraine, you'll find that low-effort, "no-brainer" meals will be much appreciated as you recover from an attack. And if you have a family to feed, having meals at the ready means less stress.

As an alternative, keep a small stockpile of restaurant and pizzeria menus from places that deliver. If the freezer is bare or you can't rely on others to do even basic meal prep, order in.

Family and Friends

If you have children, do your homework ahead of time and develop a roster of sitters, friends, and family with various availabilities, so you'll have several people to call on at any time of the day to take over for child care.

With older children, educate them about migraine so that they respect your recovery needs. Even younger children can be taught some basics about migraine disease and your need for quiet recovery in a nonfrightening manner. Have these conversations when you're feeling well so you have appropriate time for discussion and can answer any questions.

Shuttling kids to extracurricular activities or sports can become a major challenge during a migraine attack, so make a point of acquainting yourself with other team parents that you can call on for child transportation if need be. You can always return the favor when you're feeling better.

Although you may be embarrassed or self-conscious about your migraines, try to be open with family and friends. There are so many myths and misconceptions about migraine that it's important for you to educate them on the real facts behind your condition. If you feel ill equipped to handle the discussion, loan them this book, or take them to your next doctor's appointment. This knowledge should strengthen your relationship and also enable them to be a better source of support for you when you need it. It can also help you avoid hurt feelings when you have to cancel social engagements or other commitments at the last minute due to migraine. Chapter 15 has more tips for educating the people in your life about migraine disease.

When You're Away from Home

Migraines don't always happen at home, so it's important to have some strategies for adjusting your surroundings when crawling into bed isn't an option. By changing lighting, filtering outside noise, and having comfort measures close at hand, you can tackle a migraine wherever you are. When the first signs of migraine appear and you're far from home, preparation can make all the difference.

Children and adolescents who suffer from migraine should have a safe recovery place at school. Talk to the school nurse about what's available should the need arise, and how an existing space may be modified (e.g., lighting changed) to accommodate your child if necessary, and make sure that the appropriate medication and parental permission releases are in the school's hands. Turn to Chapter 12 for more information on dealing with migraines at school.

Recovery at Work

If migraine strikes in the workplace, and leaving is not an option, there are steps you can take to increase your comfort level. When possible, turn off any overhead fluorescent lighting. Since this is not an option in open office areas, retail environments, and other workspaces, carry an extra pair of comfortable sunglasses with you (a well-fitting pair that doesn't pinch the nose or ears).

If there is an office lounge or other place where you can rest until your pain relievers start to kick in, take advantage of it. When a quiet space is not available, consider resting in the back seat of your car with an eye mask on until your migraine medication takes effect.

Migraine Kits

Put together one or more migraine kits and keep one at the office, in your car, and anywhere else you spend a lot of time. Fill a tote bag with extra medications and other supplies to create a more comfortable atmosphere and minimize discomfort. These may include an eye mask, earplugs or a portable noise-conditioning unit, sunglasses, scarves to drape over lamps to diffuse light, a chemical cold pack or ice patch, and a small pillow. When you travel, keep these essentials close at hand as well. Because altitude can act as a migraine trigger in some people, this is especially important with long-distance air travel. Keep in mind that Transportation Security Administration (TSA) restrictions in airports may require some adjustments to your migraine kit. Make sure any fluids you carry, including gels or creams, are in TSA-acceptable amounts. If you have injectable migraine medication or pressurized inhalers, carrying the original prescription packaging and/or a note from your physician may prove helpful in expediting your trip through airport security. TSA regulations change over time, so check with the airport and your airline the day before you travel to make sure you're in compliance with current security guidelines.

Migraine "Hangover"

The intensity of a migraine attack can drain you both physically and mentally. Many migraineurs liken the postdromal phase, or aftereffects, of migraine to a hangover. Lingering mental cloudiness, low-grade headache, fatigue, lack of appetite, dizziness, and other symptoms can continue to affect you for several days following a migraine attack. You may also feel on edge, unsure whether or not this attack has truly finished, and on guard against a possible recurrence.

There has been limited study on the postdromal phase of migraine, and not all migraineurs experience the phenomenon. For those who do, the migraine postdrome typically lasts a day or less, although it can last longer for some people. Women report postdromal symptoms more frequently than men, and fatigue and a low-grade headache are the most commonly reported symptoms.

Brain Fog

After a migraine, you may feel as if your brain has taken a permanent vacation. Perhaps you can't find your car keys, are struggling to follow the plot line of a movie, or are unable to grasp the right word in conversation. Described by some migraineurs as "brain fog," changes in thinking and cognition during and following a migraine attack can trigger memory problems, difficulty with concentration, shortened attention span, slowed reaction time, and problems with visual/spatial processing.

 Fact

Migraineurs with aura seem to experience a greater degree of cognitive problems during and following attacks. White matter lesions (WML), visible on MRI as white spots, are also more common in migraine with aura. Further study of WMLs in migraine is needed to fully understand their significance.

The good news is that these cognitive problems are not long lasting. A number of studies have explored whether migraineurs are more likely to have long-term cognitive impairment than the general population, and no evidence of a substantial difference in brain function has been uncovered. In fact, a 2007 study published in the journal *Neurology* suggests that migraine with aura may actually be protective against cognitive decline. The study, which followed more than 1,400 subjects over the age of fifty for a twelve-year period, found those who had migraine with aura scored better on word recall tests than those without migraine.

Getting Back to Normal

The best thing you can do for yourself in the wake of a migraine is to rest and free yourself from as much stress as is practical and possible. If you're still experiencing some nonmigraine head pain, be careful not to overtreat it or a rebound headache could result. Try rest and compresses instead, and call your doctor for guidance if you can't get relief.

 Fact

Peppermint oil has been used as a medical treatment for centuries, and recent research has shown that the smell of peppermint oil may be effective in relieving tension headache. If you have a lingering postdromal headache, a sniff of peppermint oil may be a safer way to soothe the pain without risk of rebound headache.

In a day or so you should be back to normal functioning. Once you are, take a few minutes to sit down with your headache diary and note any triggers or circumstances surrounding this migraine attack, in addition to treatment notes, before they fade from memory. Look for similarities between this attack and past episodes to see if there are any patterns you and your doctor can learn from.

CHAPTER 11

Women and Migraines

WHEN IT COMES to migraine, women seem to carry most of the physical, social, and economic burden. Eighteen percent of American women are living with migraine—three times the number of men with the condition. Women perceive their migraine pain as more severe than male migraineurs, they have higher levels of migraine-related disability and associated costs, and they use more medication to treat migraine attacks. Both physiology and hormonal factors contribute to the greater prevalence of migraine in females. As women move through the stages of life from menarche through menopause, migraine follows a definite pattern and progression.

The Female Connection

Up until puberty, girls and boys experience migraine on a fairly equal footing. But once menarche (the start of menstruation) hits, girls outstrip boys three to one. In fact, up to 70 percent of women cite the onset of their period as a major migraine trigger.

This obviously indicates that hormonal changes are closely tied to migraine. But hormones aren't the sole reason that women experience more migraines than men.

Research being conducted by the UCLA Department of Neurology suggests that women have faster triggering mechanisms than men. Cortical spreading depression (CSD), a phenomenon that can be seen as waves of activity that spread across the brain's surface, has been shown to trigger both migraine headache and the frequently accompanying aura and visual symptoms. Animal studies have shown that female mice have a much lower threshold for cortical spreading depression, and that the particular brain activity leading to migraine is both easier to evoke and faster to spread in women. While there are certainly other factors involved in CSD, such as hormones, genetics, and environment, males consistently showed slower reaction and wave spreading. Further research may reveal this to be one of the chief reasons why more women than men are subject to migraines.

 Fact

The American Migraine Study II, a population-based survey of 20,000 American households sponsored by the National Headache Foundation, found that 51 percent of women who met the clinical criteria for migraine remain undiagnosed. This was higher than the rate for men, which was 41 percent.

The Hormone Connection

Female sex hormones—including estrogen and progesterone—have a major impact on how pain is mediated and perceived in women. By studying hormone levels in female migraineurs throughout the different phases of the menstrual cycle, researchers have determined that consistently high levels of estrogen and progesterone in the body are associated with a decrease in migraine frequency and severity. Conversely, migraine frequency appears to peak during the first three days of the menstrual cycle when these hormones are at their lowest levels.

 Fact

Research has shown that the genetic predisposition to migraine appears to be relatively equal in men and women. This provides further evidence that hormones play a large role in the prevalence and course of migraine in women.

It's believed that estrogen also plays a role in regulating levels of serotonin in the body, the neurotransmitter (or brain chemical) that is most associated with migraine. Blood levels of serotonin fall during a migraine; estrogen appears to increase serotonin production and the uptake of the neurotransmitter by receptors in the brain. Estrogen may also boost the pain-relief capabilities of the central nervous system.

On the other hand, estrogen supplementation in the form of birth control pills appears to increase migraine frequency and intensity in some women with menstrual migraine. Why the apparent inconsistency? Women with consistently high estrogen levels or consistently low estrogen levels appear to be less prone to migraine attacks. Researchers theorize that it is probably large fluctuations of estrogen in the blood that promote migraine. As the normal menstrual cycle and the dosing formulation of a month's supply of many birth control pill preparations produce significant hormone fluctuations in a cyclic manner, it is not hard to understand the cyclic nature of the condition in women with menstrual-related attacks or pure menstrual migraine.

 Fact

Estrogen isn't the only female sex hormone that affects migraine. Progesterone, and the chemicals it produces when it metabolizes, appears to inhibit certain pain pathways in the trigeminal nerves. Increased levels of this hormone just after ovulation seem to be associated with a decreased severity of migraine headache during this phase of the menstrual cycle.

Several studies have looked at the effect of sudden estrogen depletion in women who had been on a long-term course of estrogen supplementation. All were associated with an increase in migraine frequency once estrogen was discontinued. One study of sudden estrogen withdrawal in women undergoing in vitro fertilization found that an abrupt decrease in estrogen was associated with an 82 percent increase in migraine attacks.

Social Implications

Despite increased education and awareness of the condition, there is still a stigma associated with migraine. Women with migraine in particular may encounter stereotypes of the condition as "just a headache," "all in their head," or signs of hypochondria. It is well documented that female migraineurs experience a higher level of disability than their male counterparts, reporting longer and more severe head pain, spending more time in bed recovering, and experiencing more lost days of work and school.

In some cases, women have grown up with these false conceptions of migraine and may not seek diagnosis or appropriate care. Or, those people a woman works and socializes with and encounters throughout her day may have these preconceptions, impacting her self-esteem and quality of life. Even some health care providers may not be appropriately educated about migraines and therefore may either consciously or unconsciously perpetuate these unfounded stereotypes.

The media has not helped the situation. A 2006 review of U.S. newspaper coverage of migraine published in the journal *Mayo Clinic Proceedings* found that stories on migraine and epilepsy contained the highest prevalence of stigmatizing language (defined as wording that portrays the patient as socially undesirable or reduced in physical worth). Twenty-nine percent of migraine stories met this criteria.

 Fact

Despite an increase in available media channels, newspapers continue to be a trusted source of health care information. A survey from the Centers for Disease Control (CDC) found that newspapers and magazines are used more often as health news sources than other online and broadcast media.

The study looked at journalistic coverage of neurological diseases and conditions in the *New York Times* and eight regional newspapers with a circulation of 200,000 or more.

Interestingly, those conditions with the highest incidence of stigmatizing language garnered the least overall press coverage, perhaps demonstrating that migraine remains poorly understood by the media and by the public it serves.

Adolescence and Adulthood

Before menarche, or first menstruation, girls experience migraine at approximately the same rate as boys. But after puberty hits, female migraineurs outnumber males two to one. And the gap widens into adulthood, where women with migraine exceed men with migraine by three to one.

Given the close association between hormonal changes and migraine incidence and intensity, this phenomenon isn't surprising. The progression of migraine also follows a specific pattern within women that is closely tied to their stage of life and the hormonal changes that accompany these life periods.

Adolescence

Puberty, and specifically, the onset of menstruation, marks the beginning of migraines for many women. Approximately 10 percent of women experience their first migraine at this time of their lives. Some teens who develop migraine without aura in childhood or adolescence will "outgrow" the condition when they reach adulthood; migraine with aura seems to stay with young women (and men) throughout their lifetime.

The physical, social, and emotional changes that take place during adolescence make the added burden of migraine particularly difficult. Adolescence is a time of wanting to fit in, not stand out, and the consequences of dealing with chronic migraine—including withdrawal from social activities and missing school—are hard for even the most mature teenager to handle.

Alert

> Studies have shown that smoking increases risk of stroke seven-fold in women who have migraine with aura. If you are a female migraineur, you already have an increased risk of cardiovascular disease. Talk to your doctor about a smoking cessation program that will be compatible with your migraine treatment and slash your stroke risk.

Another challenge adolescent migraineurs face is restricted treatment options. Many migraine prophylactics and acute treatments are not well studied, and consequently not approved for use, in children and adolescents. Off-label use of migraine drugs thought to be safe for these age groups is an option. For the young woman who faces frequent migraines, dealing with a knowledgeable pediatric neurologist or headache specialist is crucial in developing an effective treatment program.

Adulthood

The frequency of migraine is at its highest between the ages of twenty-five and fifty-five for women, peaking in the early forties. That makes adulthood the most active stage of life for migraine disease. Fortunately, women are typically better equipped emotionally, physically, and financially to handle migraine in adulthood than they were during the sometimes-tumultuous period of adolescence.

Adulthood is also the time of life when building both a family and a career take center stage. Migraine can impact both. Pregnancy involves changes in treatment, covered later in this chapter, and migraine can cause disability in the workplace. The challenges of dealing with migraine on the job are covered in detail in Chapter 14.

For sexually active women, contraception choice is an important consideration for migraine treatment too. Nonpharmaceutical choices, such as an intrauterine device (IUD) or condoms, may be preferred. In women who have migraine with aura, the use of oral contraceptives could pose an increased risk of stroke or other cardiovascular events (beyond that associated with oral contraceptives in nonmigraineurs). The frequency of migraine without aura can also be impacted by oral contraceptive use. See the "Birth Control Pills" section later in this chapter for more information.

The Menstrual Migraine

Up to 12 percent of female migraineurs (and over 12 million American women) meet the clinical criteria for what is known as menstrual migraine—migraine that is specifically and exclusively tied to the menstrual cycle. This differs from menstrually related migraine, migraine that can be caused by hormonal changes related to menstruation but that also appears at other times in response to different triggers. Approximately half of women with migraine are estimated to have menstrually related migraine.

Question

My migraines happen during my period and also when I'm stressed. Do I have menstrual migraine?
Since you have at least one other identified trigger that is not associated with your menstrual cycle, it's more likely that you have menstrually related migraine.

According to the International Headache Society (IHS), the diagnostic criteria for menstrual migraine is as follows:

- Attacks occur exclusively between two days prior to or three days following the start of menstruation in at least two out of three menstrual cycles.
- Attacks do not occur at any other time of the cycle, except as noted above.
- Headache attacks last four to seventy-two hours (untreated or unsuccessfully treated)

- Headache has at least two of the following characteristics:
  - Primarily felt on one side of the head (although referred pain may be felt anywhere on the face or head)
  - Pulsating or throbbing quality
  - Moderate to severe pain intensity
  - Aggravation by or causing avoidance of routine physical activity (e.g., walking or climbing stairs)
- During headache at least one of the following occurs:
  - Nausea and/or vomiting
  - Sensitivity to light and sound (photophobia and phonophobia)
- Not attributed to another neurological or physical disorder

Most women who have diagnosed menstrual migraine do not experience aura. However, women can also experience migraine with aura that is triggered by hormonal changes related to their cycle.

Causes

Menstrual migraine is most likely tied to the drop of estrogen levels that occurs just prior to and during menstruation.

When a menstrual migraine begins after menstruation starts and is associated with dysmenorrhea (or painful cramping during menstruation), it may be caused by an increase in prostaglandin levels. Prostaglandins are the hormones that cause uterine contractions (i.e., cramping). They also set off a variety of physiological changes—including vasoconstriction and sensitization of pain receptors—that can trigger a migraine.

Essential

Cyclic prophylaxis doesn't work for everyone. Women with irregular menstrual cycles who can't accurately predict the start of their period may benefit from long-term prophylactic treatment.

Treatment

Because menstrual migraine is predictable by definition, prophylactic drugs taken around the menstrual cycle can work well. This type of treatment is called cyclic or miniprophylaxis and involves starting medication several days before menstruation and continuing into the menstrual cycle for as long as one week. Triptans appear to be highly effective for this purpose. Taken two days prior to the beginning of menses and continued throughout the cycle, triptans can reduce migraine attacks significantly.

Some nonsteroidal anti-inflammatory drugs (NSAIDs) have also proven effective as a prophylactic. One trial examining a twice-daily regimen of naproxen sodium starting seven days before menses and ending six days into the cycle helped to reduce headache pain, duration, and acute medication use. And in 33 percent of the women studied, it prevented migraine completely.

Cyclic use of transdermal estrogen patches has also proved effective in preventing menstrual migraine in some women. Use of the patch helps to facilitate consistent levels of estrogen in the body during the menstrual cycle.

Triptan drugs and analgesics such as NSAIDs can also be taken for acute treatment of migraine pain. For more on acute treatment of migraine, see Chapter 7, and for more on triptans and NSAIDs as prophylactics, see Chapter 8.

 Question

I've never had migraines, but I heard going on birth control pills can cause them! Is that true?
Yes. According to the National Institute of Neurological Disorders and Stroke (NINDS), among women who have never experienced migraines and who start oral contraceptives, the risk of migraine increases tenfold. Talk to your health care provider about the risks and benefits of oral contraceptives for you.

Birth Control Pills

Oral contraceptives containing estrogen, even those of the low-dose variety, are associated with a small but notable increased risk of stroke. Because migraine with aura is also linked to a small but notable further increased risk of stroke, the danger is compounded if a woman with the condition chooses to go on these birth control pills. This risk is yet further increased for those who smoke.

Migraine without aura is not associated with an increased stroke risk, so estrogen-based oral contraceptives may be a viable treatment choice for you if you have never experienced aura, if you are under age thirty-five, and if you have no other cardiovascular risk factors (especially smoking). A low-dose oral contraceptive may be preferred to try and avoid large fluctuations in estrogen levels during the menstrual cycle.

If You Take the Pill

Certain types of oral contraceptives that involve a week of "placebo" treatment (i.e., the inactive pills taken during the last week of the twenty-eight-day cycle) are associated with an increased incidence of migraine attacks during the placebo period. Keep a diary when you first start your course of contraceptives to see how the placebo period affects your migraine patterns.

It's possible to supplement your "placebo period" with another form of migraine treatment to prevent unwanted attacks. Your doctor can advise you on the options that exist and how they fit your health history and lifestyle needs.

If you choose to go on estrogen oral contraception because your migraines don't involve aura and you have no other cardiovascular risk factors, be vigilant. If at any point during treatment you begin to experience aura or other visual disturbances let your doctor know immediately as you may need to consider discontinuing their use.

The "Minipill"

For migraineurs who can't tolerate estrogen-based oral contraception, progestin-only pills (POP, or minipill) may be a viable choice.

The minipill works by thickening the cervical mucus (to inhibit the transport of sperm) and suppressing ovulation. However, its efficacy rate in preventing pregnancy is lower than an estrogen-containing contraceptive.

The minipill is good news for women who have migraine with aura who prefer oral contraceptives over other options. Studies to date indicate that progestin-only pills are not associated with the increased risk of stroke that estrogen-based pills are, so migraine with aura patients can safely use them, as can women over the age of thirty-five.

Migraines During Pregnancy

The first trimester of pregnancy is often associated with an increase in migraine frequency that correlates to a sudden surge in estrogen and other pregnancy-related hormones. The good news is that as hormone levels stabilize and pregnancy progresses, migraines may decrease. Almost half of pregnant migraineurs report an overall improvement in their headaches. And one study of pregnant women with migraine without aura found that 80 percent had no migraines during the third trimester of pregnancy, a finding confirmed by subsequent studies.

Of course, pregnancy presents specific challenges to the migraineur. Normal medication regimens may have to be abandoned for safety reasons, and alternatives must be found. By working with both your OB/GYN and your primary doctor for migraine, you can determine what treatments are right for you.

Safe Treatment

Medication use of any kind in pregnancy is usually a risk-versus-benefit decision. If the benefit to the mother's health outweighs any potential of risk to mother or fetus, and there are no other viable treatment options that will have similar efficacy, then a health care provider may recommend the drug.

Unfortunately, the majority of migraine medications aren't appropriate for pregnant women. They have either been proven unsafe in pregnancy through case reports or animal studies, or we simply do not have enough clinical data about their use in pregnant women to be able to make an educated "risk-versus-benefit" decision.

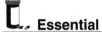
Essential

Many women with menstrual migraine will experience an improvement in the frequency of their attacks during pregnancy, usually starting toward the end of the first trimester. This migraine "honeymoon period" can even last into the postpartum period if you choose to breastfeed.

One treatment option with proven efficacy and no side effects or safety issues is biofeedback. Biofeedback is a system of monitoring your body's biological signals, such as temperature, heart rate, and muscle tension, and learning how to regulate those functions through relaxation and visualization techniques. Once you learn the skills of biofeedback, you are able to train your body to reduce migraine pain once it begins. When coupled with progressive relaxation techniques, biofeedback can be a highly effective treatment option for the first trimester and beyond. (See Chapter 7 for more information on biofeedback.)

Acupuncture may also be a safe migraine treatment alternative for pregnant and breastfeeding women. It can also have the added benefits of alleviating pregnancy-related nausea and vomiting. For more on the use of acupuncture in migraine treatment, see Chapter 9.

Fact

Unless they are a pregnancy-related treatment, most drugs aren't studied in pregnant women. Pregnant women are excluded from most clinical trials on an ethical basis, and the research that is available is in the form of animal studies and retrospective studies that analyze voluntary self-reported use of a particular drug or therapy in pregnancy after the fact.

The Postpartum Period

Both menstrual migraine and chronic migraine (with and without aura) typically resurface during the postpartum period as estrogen levels drop. An estimated 94 percent of women report that their migraines return after delivery. Women under age thirty appear to have a more rapid return to prepregnancy migraine patterns.

Alert

If you experience a severe headache following delivery, alert your doctor. While it may just be a migraine, there are several other causes of an immediate postpartum headache—including spinal headache, reaction to anesthesia, and eclampsia—that should be ruled out by your physician as a safety measure.

However, there is some evidence that breastfeeding will extend the improvement of migraine into the postpartum period for many women—another of the many health benefits of breastfeeding to mother and child. If you choose to breastfeed, keep in mind that many migraine prescription and over-the-counter drugs are contraindicated for nursing mothers because they pass into breast milk and their impact on an infant is unknown.

Migraines and Menopause

Menopause may provide migraine relief for many women. Symptoms of migraine decrease in about two-thirds of women who go through menopause naturally, but that number drops to only one-third in women who have surgical or medical menopause (i.e., hysterectomy with ovary removal).

In fact, roughly two-thirds of migraineurs who undergo surgical menopause experience worsening migraine symptoms. This may be due to the sudden drop in estrogen associated with ovary removal.

Hormone Replacement Therapy (HRT)

Hormone replacement therapy (HRT), which is sometimes prescribed to alleviate menopausal symptoms, can be either a blessing or a curse for postmenopausal female migraineurs—studies have found that HRT improves symptoms in 45 percent of women, but worsens symptoms in 46 percent.

In postmenopausal women with a history of migraine who require ERT or HRT, continuous transdermal (i.e., through the skin) treatment that provides a low and steady amount of estrogen to the body is preferred to keep hormone fluctuations to a minimum. This may be in the form of a skin patch or gel.

Large-scale, long-term studies have associated some forms of HRT with an increased risk of cardiovascular disease. The Women's Health Initiative (WHI) studied the effects of HRT use in over 27,000 women and found that estrogen plus progestin hormone replacement therapy increased the risk of heart attack, stroke, blood clots, and certain types of cancer. Estrogen-only HRT increased the risk of stroke and blood clots. While no specific studies have analyzed the use of HRT in women who have migraine with aura, because of the increased stroke risk associated with the latter it may not be the best treatment choice for postmenopausal women with the condition. If you are considering HRT as a migraine treatment, talk to your doctor about the potential risks and benefits in light of your specific health history.

Beyond Menopause

In a very small percentage of women, migraine may appear for the first time following menopause. Because of the rarity of a postmenopausal migraine diagnosis, any new chronic headache that appears after age forty-five, especially one with accompanying visual disturbances or severe debilitating pain, should be evaluated by a health care provider immediately to ensure that the symptoms are not the sign of a developing neurological illness.

CHAPTER 12

Children and Headaches

THE PAIN OF a migraine is not limited to adults. About 5 to 10 percent of children also suffer from migraines, and the overall incidence of migraine peaks in adolescence. While it is always hard for parents to see their child in pain, there are a number of steps that parents can take to help their children by effectively diagnosing and treating their child's condition.

The Youngest Patients

Children frequently complain about pain ("Mom, my foot hurts and I can't walk to take the trash out tonight." "Mom, my head hurts and I can't do my homework."). It can be difficult to know when a child is experiencing genuine pain, especially with something as seemingly intangible as a headache.

Headaches in children should always be taken seriously. Ignoring signs and symptoms can lead to more serious headache issues down the road, and can also cause resentment in your children. Treat their complaints with the respect and attention that you would treat those of your spouse or an adult friend.

Signs and Symptoms

Generally speaking, children suffer from headaches for the same reasons as adults. The types of headaches children experience are similar to those experienced by adults. However, special attention needs to be paid to the signs and symptoms that child headache sufferers commonly display.

Detective Work

Children do not tend to understand that pain is transient and can be improved, so they may be prone to omitting key details that would help in their treatment. They also do not typically keep good headache diaries or accurately report all symptoms, so figuring out the details of their specific type of headache can be a challenge.

Being a good detective can help you (and your doctor) more accurately diagnose and treat children with headache. Young children are not always aware of the cause of their pain and may have difficulty even describing it. If you suspect migraine or another recurring primary headache, you will need to learn how to ask the right questions in order for your child to aid in their diagnosis.

 Question

How common are headaches in very young children?
This is a group that is notoriously difficult to survey accurately. Children may not admit to having a headache when asked. It is much more common to have a child report that "something doesn't feel right," or "something hurts."

Getting a Diagnosis

Headache is much more commonly diagnosed in older children and teenagers. Children will typically complain of pain, either single- or dual-sided, around the front or back of the head. Beyond the basic description, though, there are several key factors in helping your child's pediatrician to diagnose their headache.

Behavior

For children of all ages, it is extremely important to look at how they are acting, in addition to whatever they can tell you about the pain they are experiencing. When young children become irritable (crying or fussy), a headache can be a culprit. Other symptoms include children deliberately avoiding bright lights or playing outside, and wanting to stay in bed under the covers (where it is dark and warm). Nausea and vomiting can also indicate migraine. All of these symptoms can also be a sign of several other significant illnesses, including pediatric brain tumors. Any headache that persists, is progressive, and is associated with changes in behavior or other physical symptoms should be evaluated by your child's pediatrician.

Especially among older children, migraine is one of the most common types of chronic headaches. Migraines affect around 10 percent of children, with the percentage rising for older children and teenagers. Migraine frequency is approximately equal between boys and girls up to the age of seven. The rate for girls begins to increase as puberty approaches, and in adolescence, females are more significantly likely to have migraines than males. When diagnosing the type of headache your child is experiencing, look for the same signals and symptoms of an adult migraineur—one-sided head pain, nausea/vomiting, and visual perception changes are the best indicators. If either parent is a migraine sufferer, it is likely that migraine may be an issue for a child who starts to complain of headache.

Occasional headaches may not signal a chronic issue. Sometimes, headache can result from fever. If your child has a cold or another illness that may come with a fever, headaches are a common side effect. If the child's pediatrician approves of the use of a fever-reducing medication such as acetaminophen, using it may also reduce this type of headache.

 Fact

Even a mild case of sunstroke can lead to headache. When playing out in the sun, make sure your child stays well hydrated and takes breaks to cool off. And if bright sunlight is a migraine trigger for your child, encourage her to wear a wide-brimmed hat or sunglasses to protect herself.

Vision Problems and Stress

Does your child frequently tell you that the blackboard at the front of the school classroom looks blurry, or does she frequently rub her eyes? When children have difficulty focusing or display other signs of a possible eyesight problem, headache can often be a result. If your child complains of transient, or short-term, visual disturbances involving blind spots and/or floating patterns, this could be a sign of a migraine aura. Talk to your pediatrician or ophthalmologist about your child's vision issues. He should be able to distinguish between a child who needs glasses and one who is experiencing the visual auras common in migraines.

Stress headaches are common in adults, but can also appear in children. Talk to your child to see if there might be a problem at school; examples of stressors in school-age children include a new school, new work that is particularly confusing, or bullying by other children. Examine your home life for anything that might be stressful—a death in the family, a new stepparent, or other change in the family structure can be very stressful to young children who don't fully understand the reason for the changes. Working to eliminate or mitigate the underlying cause of the stress can be an effective means of reducing the frequency and intensity of a child's stress headache.

Figuring Out Triggers

You know when your children go to bed, what they ate for lunch in school, and what medications they are taking. Or do you? An important step in diagnosing your child's headache is determining what their triggers actually are. When treating small children with potential migraines, parents should eliminate triggers that are within their control.

Dehydration

Dehydration can cause headaches. The definition of dehydration is excessive loss of water from the body. If a child has not been drinking regularly, typical signs will include fatigue, headache, dark-colored urine, less frequent urination, a dry-feeling mouth, and a sticky feeling inside the mouth. Children dehydrate easily, partly because of their smaller body mass, but also because they tend to get so involved in their activities that they simply forget to drink. Try preventative solutions such as having your child carry a water bottle. If they notice fewer headache signs while they are drinking more, dehydration becomes a more probable headache trigger.

Low blood sugar (hypoglycemia) is a known migraine trigger. If a child regularly skips meals due to lack of appetite, consult a pediatrician to look for other possible conditions. Some children, however, would rather play than eat, or take two bites of a meal before running off. In those cases, try engaging the child long enough to amuse them throughout a meal, providing fun-shaped child-friendly foods. In the short term, offering liquid nutritional supplements is also okay.

Foods and Smells

The same foods that trigger adult headaches can trigger headaches in children. Keep track of whether your child consumes cheese, chocolate, fried foods, or processed lunchmeats containing sodium nitrate (bologna, hot dogs, etc.) on days when headaches occur. Also keep a record of whether headache strikes on days when your child has eaten any food with monosodium glutamate; this food additive is a known trigger for migraine in adults.

Beverages can also be culprits when it comes to triggering a child's headache. Favorite children's drinks such as sodas and sports drinks can contain high amounts of caffeine. Read labels carefully on any food or drink that your child ingests regularly; even something as innocent-sounding as flavored water can contain enough caffeine to trigger a headache. Chapter 6 has more information on food and beverage triggers.

While many small children enjoy the sensation of smelling flowers on the side of the road, or brownies in the oven, for other children these scents can trigger a migraine. Common odor triggers for children include heavy perfumes, smoke, and "new car" smell. Anything strong, especially something that your child is not often exposed to, is a possible trigger.

Fact

If schedule or pickiness keeps your child from eating regular meals, try encouraging her to snack throughout the day. If migraine severity and frequency decrease, try to make sure that her blood sugar level remains consistent throughout the day in order to avoid this trigger.

Motion Sickness

A common adult headache trigger results from motion sickness. If your child notably experiences migraine symptoms after having been in a car, boat, or train, consider this as a possible trigger. The same treatments for adults can be used with children. Experiment with preventative motion-sickness medications, though you will want to avoid any that might make your child drowsy. Always check with the manufacturer, as some common Meclizine-based medications are not suitable for young children. Simple preventative measures may be effective; make sure the child does not read in the car, does not begin a long car trip on an overfull or empty stomach, and seat them in the front seat if they meet your state's height and weight requirements.

Other Triggers

Has your child been under an increased amount of stress recently? Has she been staying up too late, talking with friends on the phone or doing homework? When a child does not get enough sleep, their self-regulating body systems are thrown out of balance, and headache is a possible result. In fact, most children with headaches tend to experience them during months that schools are in session.

As with adults, childhood headaches can be triggered by certain medications. Check with your doctor and pharmacist to see if any of your child's regular or special medications list "headache" as a side effect. If this is the case, speak to your doctor to see if there might be alternate remedies available.

Does your child spend several hours playing loud music through headphones? This could easily trigger a chronic headache—and is a relatively easy trigger to test. Have your child give up the headphones for a time and see if this change makes a difference in the frequency and intensity of their headaches.

 Alert

Low lighting levels may cause eyestrain, which is a known trigger for some varieties of headache. Experiment with adjusting the lighting in your child's computer room or homework area. Replace fluorescent tubes with incandescent or compact fluorescent bulbs.

The same test applies to a child who spends hours at a time in front of either a television or computer monitor. See if breaking up the amount of "screen time" into smaller segments and eliminating a portion of the time spent sitting in front of these devices makes a difference.

Treatment Safety

Treating migraines in children follows the same basic pattern as treatment of adult migraines, though the specifics will vary considerably depending on the child's age, history, and headache specifics. The basic approach for forming a treatment plan for children with migraines includes learning to eliminate triggers, finding medications that work in the short term for acute attacks, and considering preventative medication to help ward off future migraines. Lifestyle changes that encourage stress reduction and relaxation are also important. Children and their parents should keep a headache diary and work with the child's doctors to eliminate other unlikely but possible causes, such as brain tumors or other medical conditions.

Medication

Over-the-counter pain relievers such as ibuprofen and acetaminophen are rarely helpful if taken after a migraine has begun. However, these remedies are usually safe for children and can be useful if taken at the very onset of symptoms. Because your child's digestive system will slow down if she has a migraine, liquid forms of medication will be absorbed faster.

Abortive medications, those that work to stop a migraine in its tracks, can be useful for children and fall into the same general classes as adult medications. These include triptans (sumatriptan, zolmitriptan, naratriptan) and ergotamine derivatives (ergotamine, dihydroergotamine). Chapter 7 has more information on these medications.

Some preventative medications, also known as prophylactics, are considered safe for children based on published research and anecdotal use. Prophylactics must be taken over a fairly long period of time in order for them to be effective in reducing migraine severity and frequency. The typical standard of care for using preventative medication is if the child experiences more than two headaches per week that do not respond to other remedies. Preventative medications for children generally fall into one of three categories:

- **Antiseizure medication** (valproic acid)
- **Antidepressant medication** (amitriptyline)
- **Beta-blockers** (propranolol) and **calcium channel blockers** (verapamil)

 Alert

Antidepressant drugs can cause an increased risk of suicidality (suicidal thinking and behavior) in children and adolescents. For this reason, antidepressants may not be the primary drug of choice for migraine prevention in children. If they are prescribed, the child should be closely monitored for signs of self-destructive behavior.

It's important to note that as of the publication of this book, there is no migraine treatment that is FDA approved for use in children, primarily because of the lack of rigorous controlled clinical studies on these drugs in pediatric populations.

Turn to Chapter 8 for more information on migraine prophylaxis.

Medication Avoidance

Steering clear of medications that are known to increase the likelihood of your child suffering a migraine can be a tremendous step in your child's treatment plan. Some of the more common medications on this list include but are not limited to: Cimetdine, nitroglycerin, histamines, Reserpine, Hydralazine, and Ranitidine.

Be aware that childhood headache can be the result of "analgesic rebound." If your child routinely takes large doses of over-the-counter pain medications, then suddenly stops taking them, chronic headaches can be the unfortunate result. Slow weaning off these medications may help avoid a sudden increase in migraine frequency.

Sleep and Diet

One of the simplest things a child can do to alleviate the pain of a migraine is go back to bed. Sleep removes the light and sound sensitivities that can worsen a migraine and also restores brain function to its normal levels. If your child has difficulty falling asleep, talk to her pediatrician about using a pain reliever to help alleviate the pain long enough so that she can fall asleep. Isolating dietary migraine triggers is an important way to help a child manage migraines. Common culprits, such as dairy, chocolate, and citrus, act in different ways on the body.

Essential

Other less well-known triggering foods that children tend to eat include lunchmeat, dry-roasted nuts, most flavored potato chips, bananas, and dried fruit. Keeping a headache diary will help isolate the foods and drinks that may induce migraine in your child.

Potential migraine triggers are covered in greater detail in Chapter 6.

Complementary Therapies

Because young children cannot be given some of the stronger medications that adults take for migraines, take advantage of alternative treatment options. Biofeedback and guided relaxation are two techniques that can work very well in alleviating migraine pain. Health psychologists, headache specialists, or physical therapists can provide assistance with these remedies. Older children and teenagers will typically respond better to these treatments than young children.

Try leading your child on a guided relaxation exercise, one that can help relax the body and improve a migraine. Ask your child to visualize their headache in colors, for example, or numbers. Ask them to imagine the headache fading away as if it were an ice cube placed on a hot sidewalk; visualize the pain melting as the ice melts into a pool of water. Concentrating on any sort of abstract representation will take their focus away from the pain and, in the process, will help alleviate it.

Nausea and Vomiting

Children are especially vulnerable to pangs of nausea, or that queasy feeling we all get when we think we are close to vomiting. Children are in less control of their bodies than adults, and they often do not know what to do to ease the sensation. Children have little tolerance for attempts at pacification, such as "you'll feel better soon," because "soon" can feel like an eternity to a child.

Vomiting is understandably unpleasant, and the physical and psychological stress brought on by vomiting can worsen the pain of a migraine episode. Treating the nausea and vomiting that are often associated with migraine can be a challenge with children, but there are several effective remedies available. For small children, dehydration quickly becomes an issue. Look for warning signs such as fewer wet diapers or trips to the bathroom, lethargy, fussiness, and a sunken fontanel in infants. If dehydration becomes severe and cannot be corrected at home, the child may require hospitalization.

Simple Remedies

Ginger has been used for centuries to treat nausea associated with gastrointestinal upset, pregnancy, and a host of other ailments. Offer your child a cup of ginger ale, or make a fast ginger tea by steeping a piece of peeled ginger root in hot water for several minutes. There are a variety of foods and snacks containing ginger, including ginger candy and ginger lollipops, but a simple drink will be absorbed faster (and has a greater chance of staying down).

Cold, carbonated, clear beverages are soothing to a nauseous child. Until your child is no longer vomiting, avoid solid foods (or limit them to simple starches such as crackers or bread). If you think your child is becoming dehydrated, offering a pediatric rehydrating drink may help her feel better faster.

Dehydration generally makes nausea worse. Encourage your child to drink any clear fluids—water, broth, or clear soft drinks are well tolerated and may help the nausea abate faster. If she refuses liquids, offer popsicles (avoid citrus flavors, though, as the acidic content may prove too challenging for an upset stomach).

Medication

Abortive medications such as triptans can be very helpful in alleviating nausea associated with migraine. There are a variety of other antinausea drugs on the market, some of which may prove useful to your child. One of the most common is Promethazine (Phenergan), which is available as a syrup. Promethazine is an antihistamine, but also has antinausea effects and can be helpful in preventing motion sickness. It is not safe to give to a child younger than two years old. It is also sometimes used as a sedative, and often causes drowsiness.

Other prescription medicines used to treat nausea include trimethobenzamide (Tigan), metoclopramide (Reglan), and prochlorperazine (Compazine). All are prescription medications, and some may cause drowsiness. Trimethobenzamide is an antinausea medicine that blocks one of the chemical messengers in the brain from stimulating nausea and vomiting. It is safe for children but should not be used to treat vomiting in children if the vomiting is due to an unknown cause. If the vomiting is associated with Reyes syndrome, a serious disease that affects the brain, liver, and other organ systems, trimethobenzamide could make the syndrome worse.

Essential

Note that if your child is vomiting up everything she eats or drinks, oral medication will not do much good. Most antinausea medications are available from your pediatrician as suppositories, and these tend to work quickly.

Metoclopramide works by stimulating the stomach and intestines and aids in moving food more quickly through the digestive system. It also has been proven effective in stimulating the brain to control nausea. Though metoclopramide has not been officially approved for use in children under fifteen years old, it has been used successfully on children under the close supervision of a doctor. Prochlorperazine is a phenothiazine, and blocks the brain chemical dopamine in order to help treat nausea. It should not be used in children who are under twenty pounds or less than two years old, or on children who are having surgery.

Hospitalization

In some cases, as with adults, children with migraines need to be hospitalized. If your child is vomiting to the point where she appears lethargic and dehydrated, for example, intravenous fluids may be required.

A trip to the hospital can be an extremely frightening time for a child. Depending on your child's age and her understanding of the situation, keep her informed and instruct her doctors to do the same.

Bring your child's health records, as everyone has a tendency to forget simple facts (the name of the child's doctor, her last dose of prescription medication, etc.) in times of stress. Help your child to stay calm and explain that the doctors are there to help. This is the best thing you can do to help her recover from the migraine and from the experience of being hospitalized.

School and Migraines

Migraine headaches do not occur at a time that is convenient. They can strike at just about any time, including when a child is at school. This can be particularly challenging for a parent of a young child. Make sure that school staff are aware of your child's condition and know how to appropriately and quickly take action to soothe her pain. Minimizing triggers in the classroom and school environment is also critical to minimizing the frequency of your child's migraine episodes.

Triggers at School

If your child's headache regularly develops as soon as he gets home from school, but not on the weekends, consider a visit to the ophthalmologist. It is entirely possible that your child is suffering from eyestrain caused by poor vision, and the eyestrain mainly occurs when the child is reading a whiteboard at the other end of the classroom. One quick supportive measure is to request that your child be moved to the front of the class temporarily, or that the teacher write with a darker-colored ink for a few days. If fewer headaches result, eyestrain is a good possibility.

Many parents go to great lengths to pack healthy lunches for their school-age children. However, if your child regularly eats lunch in the cafeteria, you may have little (or no) control over what she is eating there. If she dines on cheese pizza and chocolate milk every day and comes home with a headache, try sending her to school with a dairy-free and chocolate-free lunch for a week and see if her headaches abate. If the child must eat school lunch, instruct her to opt for salads, whole grain breads, and other foods with less of a chance to trigger a migraine.

Getting Help

If your child's headaches become debilitating, they will need help from the school. Educating your child's teacher, principal, and school nurse can be a huge step toward making them aware of the fact that your child may require their assistance. Have a proactive meeting with these key individuals, during which time you make them aware of your child's migraine early warning signs and symptoms. Leaving abortive prescription medication with the school nurse will be a comfort to your child, should the medication become necessary. It can also be helpful to leave ginger ale, quick-freeze popsicles, eyeshades, or other supportive remedies with the nurse in a special bag with your child's name on it. Make sure the school has all of your contact information, so that you can be reached quickly if your child needs you.

Missing Class

Children with migraine may miss school time, depending on the frequency and duration of your child's headaches. While preventative treatment can help cut down on missed class time, doctor's visits, hospitalization, and other treatments may require that your child is occasionally absent. A recent study of 970,000 school-aged migraineurs found that they missed 329,000 school days every month.

Keeping up with missed schoolwork is imperative, and not only to make sure your child does not fall behind. Migraine headaches will make your child feel that she's different and that she stands out from her classmates; if she misses assignments or projects due to her headaches, she may feel like even more of an outsider. Help her to maintain friendships with other children who can help her make up class work or bring her missed assignments.

Note that school can, in and of itself, be a migraine trigger. The stress of new teachers, a new school, difficult classmates, or any number of other factors can contribute to migraine. Once you've identified potentially triggering sources at school, work with both your child and school faculty to minimize their influence or remove them from your child's day.

 Fact

Sometimes, a factor at the school could be a triggering factor for your child's migraine. Work with educators and school staff to uncover hidden triggers such as overhead fluorescent lights, teachers wearing particularly strong perfume, or pizza day in the cafeteria.

Helping Kids Cope

Adults with migraines realize and understand that some amount of lifestyle modification is usually required if they want to be able to better control migraine frequency and intensity. Children, however, may not be capable of understanding the need to change anything about their daily life. Without adequate explanation and support, the very idea of change is frightening to many children, and parents must approach the subject carefully.

Dietary Changes

If chocolate, for example, is determined to trigger migraines in your child, eliminating it may be required. What do you say to your five-year-old the next time he asks for his favorite treat? Telling him that chocolate "makes him sick" can quickly lead to sadness on your child's part or, in worse cases, the urge to secretly binge on chocolate when his parents are not looking. Simply no longer having chocolate in the house may be a better solution. If your other children insist on having chocolate, encourage them to indulge at a friend's house.

Another solution is to provide an alternative special treat. For example, if the other children in the house love pizza but it triggers your son's migraines, allow him to have ice cream on pizza day.

When the child is older, instruction in avoiding foods that may trigger a migraine is appropriate.

Sleep and Sun

Lack of sleep is a migraine trigger for many children. Fortunately, it is one with a fairly easy countermeasure: get more sleep! Enforce a consistent bedtime, and prepare your child's room to be optimal for sleeping. Keeping the room at a cool temperature, installing shades or blinds to darken the room, and providing your child's favorite sheets and blankets will all encourage good sleeping habits. On the other hand, children with migraine frequently have difficulty with sleep, especially getting to sleep. If this is a consistent problem, despite all efforts, consult your doctor.

Similarly, overexposure to sun triggers many headaches, but the solution need not be a life led completely indoors. Sun exposure can be mitigated by your child wearing a shaded cap and sunscreen, having adequate water to drink, sitting under a beach umbrella, and spending most time outdoors when the sun is not at its peak.

CHAPTER 13

Men and Migraines

MIGRAINE HEADACHES AFFECT a significant portion of the population, roughly 15 percent. The good news for men is that about three times as many women as men suffer from migraines. The bad news for men, however, is that these percentages are very little comfort when someone is under attack from a severe headache. While men are significantly less likely to be migraineurs, the reality is that many men do suffer from migraines. Many of the treatment options for men and women are the same, but there are some distinctly male issues relating to chronic headaches.

The Silent Minority

Because migraine is often seen as a "women's issue," male sufferers rarely get the attention, or the research effort, that goes into female migraine. However, male sufferers require abortive and preventative treatment in the same manner that women do. Migraine occurs in men who have relatives with migraines, and men and women have similar migraine triggers.

It is never wise to ignore migraine pain, although many men do it. Men in American society are traditionally expected to "tough it out" more than women. They tend to seek less treatment for headache and, when they do, they tend to follow up with fewer specialists for migraine pain.

While working through the pain does allow people to maintain some amount of normalcy in their routine, quality of life will ultimately be affected in the presence of persistent, spontaneous pain. Job performance can suffer, as can one's relationships with friends and family. The longer head pain is ignored, the longer it may take to diagnose and treat it. Longer absences from work mean risking losing one's job, so ultimately it saves time, money, and personal well-being to pay attention to headaches as they occur.

 Fact

Migraines are thought to be triggered by cortical spreading depression, or CSD, a wave of electrical activity in the brain. Animal studies have demonstrated that in males, the threshold for triggering CSD is much higher than that for females—about three times higher—perhaps suggesting an explanation for the migraine gender gap.

Silent Migraine

One migraine diagnosis more common in men than women is a phenomenon known as the "silent migraine," also called an acephalgic or migraine aura without headache. This specific type of migraine episode is characterized by visual disturbances, aura, slurred speech and other symptoms, but generally does not present with a headache. Men are considerably more likely to suffer from this than women.

While silent migraine is typically benign and not linked to any serious health consequences, it can disrupt work and social activities and impact quality of life. Silent migraine is notoriously difficult to diagnose. Without the hallmark symptom of the headache, silent migraine is often confused with a variety of other neurological and health problems, including stroke, Ménière's disease, and hypoglycemia. It has also been shown that a large number of migraine sufferers (as many as 20 percent) have had at least one silent migraine episode.

The best way for men to accurately have an acephalgic migraine diagnosed is with a solid medical history. It is crucial for men to keep an accurate headache diary that records all symptoms, as acephalgic migraine diagnosis relies on accurate notation of symptoms. Writing down the symptoms, time it occurred, and pain scale can be immensely useful to a general practitioner or specialist because a continued diary enables them to see patterns.

Ophthalmic Migraine

Another type of migraine that occurs disproportionately in young men is called an ophthalmic migraine. This migraine variation is related to what is called a retinal or ocular migraine. The ocular migraine is a type of migraine that presents with visual anomalies where there is eye pain and temporary blindness. There may or may not be a headache associated with an eye migraine.

Chapter 1 has more information on silent and ophthalmic migraine variants.

 Alert

The retinal blindness from an ophthalmic migraine generally resolves fairly quickly, usually within an hour, but requires the same treatment as a typical migraine. Migraineurs who encounter ophthalmic migraines should always consult an ophthalmologist to make sure there is no other medical reason for vision problems.

Migraine or Cluster Headache?

Cluster headaches may be considered a type of migraine, but there are several important distinctions. As described in depth in Chapter 2, cluster headaches come in episodes, varying from a week to a year, while most migraines consist of a single episode. In addition, cluster headaches belong more to the realm of men. While less than 0.5 percent of the population suffers from cluster headaches, nearly 80 percent of those cases consist of men. Women can also have cluster headaches or cluster migraines, but they are in the minority.

Distinctions

How can men tell the difference between cluster headaches and frequent migraines? Because men are much more likely to suffer from cluster headaches than women, the temptation is to jump to a diagnosis of cluster headache. However, because some treatments for these types of headaches are not the same, it is critical to obtain a correct diagnosis.

Generally, the diagnosis must be made with the help of a detailed headache diary. Taking note of when headaches occur, and for how long, can be key in differentiating a cluster headache from a traditional migraine. Cluster headaches tend to appear in the middle of the night, for example, whereas traditional migraines do not. Cluster headaches can be gone in less than an hour, where a migraine generally lasts for much longer without the aid of abortive medication. Migraines often have warning signs and symptoms, where cluster headaches often appear to come "out of nowhere," and they often arrive with a vengeance.

Essential

The location of headache pain tends to differ with clusters and migraines. Men experiencing cluster headaches often describe pain that occurs either behind or around one eye. Cluster headache pain is generally considered sharp, or stabbing. Migraine pain tends to be duller and more throbbing, and often spreads to the front or back of the head.

Ancillary symptoms are another important diagnostic tool. If a man suffers from headaches frequently and tends to have accompanying facial pain, particularly on one side or the other, cluster headaches may be more likely. Oftentimes, cluster headaches are accompanied by sinus headache, including nasal congestion, watering eyes, and facial puffiness. These symptoms tend to correlate less often with migraines.

Treatment

Acute cluster headache treatment overlaps with acute migraine treatment; standard therapy includes triptan medication. There are also acute treatments that work more specifically on cluster headaches but are less effective on migraines. Intranasal lidocaine or capsaicin, for example, has been shown to be more effective on cluster headaches than migraine. In addition, oxygen therapy is a highly effective treatment for cluster headaches.

Cluster headaches may respond to some of the same preventative treatments as migraine headaches. Ergotamines are taken in the hour or so before a headache is expected to land with full force, and they work well for nighttime use. Valproic acid takes several days to work but is also effective as a prophylactic. Other remedies that are not necessarily beneficial for migraineurs can work well for cluster headaches. Prednisone is an oral steroid that works quickly, but has a variety of side effects such as weight gain and hyperglycemia (high blood sugar). Lithium is also highly effective in stopping cluster headache, but it also is associated with an array of troublesome side effects, including tremor, nausea, fatigue, weight gain, and potential kidney and thyroid problems.

The success of treatment can, in and of itself, be a factor in making a correct diagnosis. If oxygen therapy is successful, for example, there is increased evidence for the presence of a cluster headache as opposed to a traditional migraine.

Testosterone and Male Headache

Some research suggests that testosterone therapy may help alleviate the pain of migraine and cluster headaches. A 2006 study by the Cleveland Clinic Foundation described the relationship of both cortisol and testosterone to cluster headaches.

A few important terms:

- **Cortisol**, known as the "stress hormone," is a corticosteroid hormone that is produced by the adrenal cortex. Cortisol increases blood pressure and blood sugar, and has a wide array of effects on the body's organ systems.

- **Testosterone** is a steroid hormone secreted by both males and females; in men, it is released by the testes and the adrenal gland, and is responsible for supporting secondary male sexual characteristics.
- **DHEA** is a hormone that is secreted by the adrenal gland and is a precursor to the sex hormones androgens and estrogens.
- **Pregnenolone** is a steroid hormone that is the precursor for all other corticosteroids.
- **Melatonin**, known as the "sleep hormone," is a hormone that is synthesized in the pineal gland that helps regulate the body's sleep cycle.

This study demonstrated the possibility that inadequate production of cortisol and testosterone were seen in sufferers of cluster headaches. Other studies have found similar results: patients who are diagnosed with cluster and migraine headaches tend to have lower-than-standard levels of total testosterone, DHEA sulfate, and pregnenolone. Similarly, both men and women with migraines have been shown to have lower blood levels of magnesium and melatonin than individuals who do not suffer from migraines. Treatment possibilities include a range of hormone and steroid therapies. See Chapter 20 for more information on future migraine treatments.

 Fact

Estrogen and migraine in women have been shown to have a direct correlation. Menstruating women experience more migraines than younger girls, and migraines are frequently triggered by the decrease of estrogen that occurs during a woman's menstrual cycle. Estrogen supplementation has been used with some success in treating menstrual migraine.

Testosterone in Women

Decrease in testosterone is also shown to be a factor in women who experience migraines. Testosterone typically declines in females as they approach menopause; it can also occur in women who have had their ovaries removed. Research shows that migraine prevalence is increased for women who, for either reason, have very low testosterone.

See Chapter 11 for more on women and migraines.

Heart Disease Connection

Migraine has been linked to an increased incidence of cardiovascular events, including heart attack and stroke, in men. A heart attack, or acute myocardial infarction (MI), occurs when blood flow to the heart is blocked, and the heart receives inadequate blood and oxygen, resulting in heart muscle death. A stroke, or cerebrovascular accident (CVA), is a loss of brain function that occurs when the blood supply to the brain is interrupted.

The link between heart disease and migraine in men was revealed in 2007 when researchers from Brigham and Women's Hospital and Harvard University published a long-term, large-scale analysis of male migraineurs involved in the Physicians' Health Study.

The Physicians' Health Study

The Physicians' Health Study is an ongoing, long-term study launched in 1982 to address areas of men's health research. The study subjects consist of more than 20,000 male doctors between the ages of forty and eighty-four with no prior history of heart disease or cancer. These men are surveyed annually for health data, providing researchers with an important resource for longitudinal (or long-term) men's health studies.

The Brigham researchers found that approximately 1,500 of the Physician's Health Study subjects experienced migraines, and survey results from 2006 showed that the male migraineurs had a significantly increased risk of heart attack and stroke. The chances of experiencing serious cardiovascular problems in the migraine population were increased by 24 percent over the general population, and their chances of a heart attack were 42 percent greater than nonmigraineurs.

Women who have migraines are also more likely to experience stroke and other cardiovascular problems; see Chapter 19 for more information on cardiovascular comorbidities. The connection between migraine sufferers and those with cardiac events is extremely interesting, as it appears that migraine could be a marker for potential future cardiac problems. Whether this knowledge can aid in the ultimate prevention of migraine or cardiac events is an area that requires substantial further research.

Overcoming Stereotypes

One of the largest issues surrounding men and migraines is the social stigma surrounding the men who experience them. Men are stereotyped as leaders and role models. Dating back to ancient civilizations, men have been the hunters and food gatherers, the head of the household who never falters. A man succumbing to a simple headache? Never!

The reality, though, is that migraines are not simple headaches. They are complex events that attack multiple systems in the human body. Neither their presentation nor treatment is simple, in either men or women, but men face an extra challenge: in addition to having to battle the migraine itself, men have to fight the cultural stereotypes against their needing help in the first place.

Extra Efforts

Male sufferers of migraines therefore have an additional emotional component to their pain. Men have to work harder than women to convince doctors, specialists, and even homeopathic practitioners of the validity of their migraine. Because migraines are less frequent in men, it often takes longer for men than for women to receive a diagnosis of migraine. Men can also succumb to frustration stemming from not being believed by family members and coworkers. Migraine can be a painful and exhausting condition, for both men and women, and men need to be aware of this social stigma as they reach out for support.

Standing Strong

Contrary to popular belief, men do not have "all the answers" any more than women do. Women frequently ask a doctor, "Why do I suffer from migraines? What is the cause?" Men are less likely to ask this question of their medical practitioners but are no less deserving of an answer. Men need to keep the same headache diaries as women, and be equally proactive in helping to form their diagnoses.

Alert

Successful treatment requires successful diagnosis, and it is imperative that men break down barriers to their own emotional and physical well-being by learning to ask the right questions concerning their health. Rather than remaining stoic and silent, men must tell the doctor about all symptoms, regardless of their apparent relevance.

Men may also have trouble admitting to their doctors that they have a condition that requires medical attention. Men don't usually complain to doctors about symptoms that they feel they can live with and, as a result, may not tell their doctor about the symptoms that are most troubling. Simply having migraines does not commit a man to a future with migraines. The more open he can be with the physician, the greater the chance that the patient and doctor, together, can arrive at a solid diagnosis and treatment plan.

Special Issues

Certain issues of migraine management differ between the genders. While there is overlap in treatment, identifying the optimal treatment has different requirements for men and women. It would benefit men to be aware of these requirements so that a fast and accurate diagnosis can be made.

"Male" Triggers

While certain foods can be migraine triggers for men and women equally, men may be more likely to indulge in some triggering foods than women. Red wine, other forms of alcohol, and cigarette smoke are known triggers for migraine. Statistically speaking, college-age men drink more than twice as much alcohol as college-age women. Among older adults, males consume about 40 percent more alcohol than women. In this respect, male migraineurs would do well to moderate their alcohol consumption when it is determined to be a triggering factor for migraine.

Essential

Once migraine triggers are identified, men need to be willing to make lifestyle changes. Locating the triggers is not enough. Men with migraines must work to actively eliminate triggers from their daily routines.

If smoking is found to be a migraine trigger, men need to be willing to remove themselves from smoky environments and, if necessary, from people who bring smoke into their lives. Men are also more likely to be smokers themselves—a 2004 study by the U.S. Centers for Disease Control (CDC) found a median smoking rate of 23.2 percent across forty-nine states for men, as compared to a 19.2 percent median smoking rate for women. But while the prevalence of smoking is greater in men, women appear to have a more difficult time kicking the habit. A 2001 review of over 100 smoking cessation research studies published in *CNS Drugs* found that men had a greater success rate in quitting smoking than women, and also tended to benefit more from nicotine replacement therapy than women did.

Seeking Treatment

One common trap that male migraineurs tend to fall into is the idea that they can treat themselves. "I know I have a migraine and I know how to treat it" is a common attitude among male migraine sufferers. Some men tend to refrain from making and keeping doctor's appointments for anything that is not broken or bleeding, but in the case of migraine headache, avoidance will not lead to absolution. For starters, most abortive and preventative migraine medications are prescription-only, so by avoiding a trip to the doctor, men are denying themselves some of medical science's strongest treatment options.

Furthermore, knowledge of migraine triggers and treatments is constantly changing. What might have worked for a migraineur when the migraines first started occurring twenty years ago may no longer be the best treatment option. In addition, it is always possible for people to build up a tolerance to some of the medications used in the treatment and prevention of migraines. When drug tolerance occurs, the medications taken daily will become less and less effective, meaning that new methods of treatment become critical.

Accepting Treatment

While men are typically willing to swallow a pill or use a nasal spray, many are wary of such "touchy-feely" treatments as biofeedback and craniosacral therapy. They often involve a relinquishment of boundaries and can leave the recipient feeling somewhat emotionally exposed. The more that men can let themselves accept nontraditional therapies, the more options become available in the treatment and prevention of migraine.

An important realization for men with migraines is the apparent duality of their migraine and treatment. Many migraine triggers can actually double as remedies, depending on the extent, duress, and condition. Women tend to have an easier time accepting this, and they are more willing to explore treatment options.

Exercise can trigger migraine under several cases: intense, sudden exercise that begins with no warm-up period, exercise with low blood sugar, or exercising while dehydrated can all be contributing factors to a migraine. Studies show that women tend to be willing to start a slow, moderate exercise plan and follow the rules of remaining hydrated. Men, on the other hand, have a tendency to jump into exercise at full velocity, even if they had not exercised in years, thus increasing their risk factors for triggering a migraine.

If a headache results, men tend to cease their workouts completely. Women tend to evaluate the situation, make adjustments, and try again. In this particular case, men can learn from the example women set: research, modify, and repeat. Never be afraid to fail in your attempt to find a working treatment plan for migraines. The more you experiment, the more likely you are to find a treatment plan that works well.

 Fact

Exercise is an important example of an activity that can both trigger and relieve migraines. Regular, moderate exercise is often seen to reduce the frequency and severity of migraines because it stimulates the release of endorphins, natural painkillers produced by the body in times of pain and exertion.

Depression

In addition to the perceived stigma of suffering from a chronic disease like migraine, men are often susceptible to depression resulting from their diagnosis. Many men tend to feel ashamed or embarrassed by any perceived weakness. In many male cultures, illness is equated with weakness. Men who see themselves as weak can, over time, become depressed and reluctant to seek help for their condition. Adding to this depression is the fact that, without treatment, migraines can become debilitating to the point where the migraineur might miss school, work, social functions, and major life events, thus sowing the seeds for further depression.

Depression is treatable through behavioral therapy, medication, lifestyle changes, and other therapeutic measures. Depression related to migraine pain may be alleviated by seeking appropriate treatment promptly. If men are able to step outside of their perceived guilt or shame to speak to a medical professional about their condition, they are already well on the way to living a happier and more fulfilling life.

CHAPTER 14

Living Life

LIFE WITH MIGRAINE is, simply put, not the same as life before a migraine diagnosis. Receiving a diagnosis of migraine, and starting a treatment plan, have an undeniable affect on one's daily routines and habits. However, that does not mean that a similar quality of life cannot be achieved with a migraine-friendly lifestyle. An excellent strategy to achieve a state of health and happiness is to make small, gradual changes in routines and activities. By reducing or eliminating migraine triggers, and recognizing a few fundamental facts about living with migraines, migraineurs can lead complete and fulfilling lives.

Healthy Sleep Patterns

There has long been a known association between sleep and migraine. Generally speaking, too little sleep or too much sleep (in the absence of any other factor) will not trigger a migraine. A full eight hours a night, or as little as five to six hours, may not trigger a migraine. However, disruption to an established sleep pattern can be a primary trigger.

Suppose someone is used to going to bed at 11 P.M., rising at 6 A.M. and eating breakfast at 7 A.M. every day. After a particularly late night, the person goes to sleep at 1 A.M. and rises at noon the following day. A migraine develops steadily over the course of the day.

What might have happened to cause the migraine? For starters, our friend got four more hours of sleep than she was accustomed to getting. Irregular sleep patterns are a known migraine trigger. Note, also, that the person delayed the first meal of the day by at least five hours. Low blood sugar, resulting from fasting in this case, is another potential trigger.

Causes of Disruption

Change in sleep patterns can result from a number of different events. Women tend to sleep poorly during certain points in their menstrual cycle. Good sex (or bad sex) can affect how long it takes to fall asleep. Having a cold or respiratory infection changes the quality and length of the sleep cycle as well. Emotional issues, such as nightmares or problems at work, can result in the inability to relax enough to fall into a deep sleep. Room temperature, lightness level, and other environmental factors can all contribute to a night of tossing and turning.

Certain medications can affect sleep patterns. Common culprits include antidepressants, antihistamines, antiarrhythmics (medications that treat heart rhythm problems), and anything containing caffeine.

 Fact

Many people will take a sleeping pill in an effort to assure a full night's rest, but some are addictive and may have a rebound effect. Any of a variety of medical conditions, or secondary pain from an injury, can also ruin a perfectly good night's sleep.

Research has shown that up to half of all migraine sufferers also have disturbances in their sleep patterns. It is a vicious cycle; lack of sleep leads to a migraine, and once someone has a migraine, falling asleep can become more difficult. The perturbed sleep cycle is therefore continued, making it harder to recover from the migraine completely.

What is interesting about sleep and migraines is that, in addition to being a trigger, sleep is one of the best remedies for migraine. Falling asleep, even for an hour, commonly eliminates migraine symptoms. However, migraine sufferers also frequently fall victim to insomnia. Either the pain of the migraine, or the stress of feeling like one must fall asleep to ameliorate or prevent a headache, can easily lead to a virtual inability to fall and stay asleep.

Solutions

Promote healthy sleep patterns by establishing rules and abiding by them. Create a bedtime routine where going to sleep at a certain time, and rising at a certain time, become daily habits. Aim for a reasonable amount of sleep (somewhere in the neighborhood of eight hours) every night. If falling asleep proves difficult, explore alternative methods first. Cold gel packs placed over the eyes work wonders for many migraineurs. Try practicing yoga, playing soft music, and using progressive relaxation techniques to put the mind and body equally at rest. A warm bath before bed can be relaxing, as can a cup of tea or any soothing (noncaffeinated) beverage.

 Alert

Easing one's emotional state can go a long way toward assuring sound sleep. Leave work disputes at work, and try to avoid conflict at home in the hours before bedtime. A peaceful evening is a good way to begin the night.

Exercise—Why It Works

Exercise plays much the same role with migraines as sleep. When done in an appropriate and consistent manner, exercise can be a wonderful preventative tool for warding off headaches. However, it can also be a primary migraine trigger.

Endorphins

Moderate aerobic exercise is beneficial to many aspects of our lives, and not only to assure us of looking good in a bathing suit. Getting a good workout releases endorphins, the painkillers naturally produced by our bodies. These endorphins serve multiple purposes in the body, but in this case, they can help relieve the pain of a migraine.

On the other hand, any major change in routine can trigger a migraine. When it comes to exercise, a new routine that is begun abruptly has the potential to cause a headache. It is generally thought that migraineurs have a more sensitive neurological system that makes them more susceptible to changes in routine, and exercise is no exception.

 Fact

Weightlifting with particularly heavy weights, for example, frequently causes muscle spasms. These spasms can lead to headaches, even for those who do not typically have migraines, but the likelihood is greater for someone already predisposed to chronic headaches.

Certain types of exercise may be more prone to triggering migraines than others. Remember that secondary factors related to exercise can also trigger migraine; exercising with low blood sugar, or failing to stay hydrated while exercising, are prime conditions for winding up with a headache.

Solutions

A good way to begin an exercise routine is slowly and gradually. Begin with a modified portion of the anticipated workout and exercise at a very low intensity for the first few days. Some physicians recommend starting an exercise regime with as little as ten to fifteen minutes a day. As the body becomes fitter and more accustomed to exercise, gradually increase the duration and intensity of workouts. For best results try working with a personal trainer, someone who can monitor progress and work with you to create an exercise plan.

Essential

Most forms of exercise are considered beneficial for those who suffer from migraines. Everything from jogging and walking to cycling, swimming in an indoor pool, yoga, and Tai Chi can be highly beneficial forms of exercise. Breaks in routine are difficult for migraine sufferers, so it is recommended to exercise on a daily basis.

Be aware that headache as a result of exercise does not necessarily mean that the exercise triggered a migraine. Based on research conducted at the Montefiore Medical Center in New York, it has been seen that some patients who had headaches only during exercise actually suffered from heart disease. This somewhat rare condition, dubbed "cardiac headache," is seen mostly in people over fifty years old who display other risk factors for heart problems. When in doubt, talk to a physician.

Sex and Intimacy

"Not tonight, dear, I have a headache" is perhaps the most common and clichéd excuse for bedroom boredom. The reality is that, when in the throes of a major migraine attack, most people do not want to be touched, bounced, jostled, or otherwise engaged in physical intimacy. Putting aside the issue of sex, many migraineurs prefer to let the migraine pass while they are in a dark room, isolated from other people. Intimacy, as well as sex, is put on hold.

Just Saying Yes

For others, though, sex plays an interesting role in the life of a migraineur. While enduring an acute migraine attack is a surefire way to kill desire, some research indicates that migraine sufferers may actually have higher levels of sexual desire than people who do not have frequent headaches. A 2006 Wake Forest study found that self-reported levels of sexual desire among migraineurs were 20 percent higher than those of tension headache sufferers. This may be due to the role that the neurotransmitter serotonin plays in both migraine and libido. Migraineurs are thought to have a deficiency of serotonin, while high levels of the neurotransmitter are associated with decreased sex drive.

A handful of small studies have indicated that orgasm can actually relieve migraine pain for some people. This may be due to the increased levels of endorphins and corticosteroids that are released with orgasm, two substances that may have an analgesic action on migraine pain.

Just Saying Maybe

The bad news: in some people, orgasm can cause a migraine rather than relieve one. One type of migraine, called an "exertional migraine," can result from any sort of strenuous activity. Exertional migraines can come with or without aura and may last as long as twenty-four hours. They are more common in women than men, and the pain typically affects both sides (or front and back) of the head. Those who find themselves with exertional migraines may want to refrain from sexual activity until the migraine has receded. Visiting a physician is also recommended, as postcoital headaches could potentially have other causes.

 Fact

Sex also releases serotonin, the brain chemical that sends "feel-good" messages to your body. Low levels of serotonin have historically been observed in migraine sufferers; migraine treatment with ergotamine derivatives affects serotonin levels.

In an effort to avoid a migraine trigger, some migraineurs may stop having sex altogether. Let your health care provider know if fear of migraine is causing you to avoid sexual activity. Preventative medications, or a change of your current migraine treatment regimen, may be in order. It is also important not to confuse sex with intimacy. While some relationships can survive without sex, few will withstand the test of time without intimacy. Both partners in a relationship need to feel valued, respected, and special to each other; intimacy is an important tool in separating your partner from everyone else in your life. Consider nonsexual ways of remaining intimate, or work alternate sexual activities into your lovemaking life.

Migraines in the Workplace

Whether one strikes at home, at school, in the office, or in the car, there is no good time to have a migraine. Having a migraine at home is one of the least inconvenient spots, since all of the comforts, medications, remedies, and other tools to fight migraines are generally located there.

Managing Migraines at Work

When migraine symptoms begin at work, the migraineur has decisions to make. Should she continue working or inform her superiors and go home for the day? Does she have enough sick time saved up to afford to leave, or does she need to use a vacation day? Does her office have a place where she could lie down and rest if necessary?

While pushing through a migraine that appears during the workday may seem unavoidable, sometimes it is simply not possible. The combination of light sensitivity, aura, dizziness, and a throbbing head can easily render the workday a complete loss. In such cases, migraine sufferers have no choice but to go home, thereby presenting a cost to the employer.

Taking Its Toll

With enough episodes of missed time on the job, employers may (either consciously or subconsciously) start leaving a migraineur out of key work decisions. She might be overlooked for promotions or not given opportunities that are presented to other employees. Her own productivity may start to decline, with enough missed days, and she will almost certainly be left out of the loop on important occurrences. While such discrimination may be illegal, it can still happen, and its effects can be hard to erase. The solution lies mainly in having an understanding employer who can make reasonable accommodations for migraine attacks that occur during the workday.

Unfortunately, there may be a stigma in some offices about people with migraines. Migraine is a hidden disability, and because migraineurs "look fine," coworkers and supervisors may not provide the support and accommodations necessary during a migraine attack. Migraineurs may be perceived as receiving unfair advantages not provided to other employees and may even be accused of feigning illness or avoiding work responsibilities.

Some migraineurs have been accused of alcohol abuse or drug dependence. Someone with a migraine may walk around, indoors or out, with dark sunglasses to shield them from bright lights. They may be seen or heard vomiting in the restroom, might have slurred speech or walk with a veering motion, or might be forced to leave work early. All of these signs may be misinterpreted as drug or alcohol related by an uneducated coworker.

Being Proactive

Proper and timely education of coworkers and superiors is usually the best defense for those who must work with a migraine. Start by explaining that migraines are a disease, not simply a "really bad headache." Those with migraines should not try to hide their pain and symptoms, as such efforts will likely only further coworkers' confusion.

Where possible, reduce triggers in the office. Turn off fluorescent lights that cause sensitivity. Reduce eyestrain by getting frequent eye exams, using antiglare screen coatings, and making sure never to work on a computer in a completely dark room. Ask coworkers to avoid wearing strong perfumes and request to be moved away from smokers—secondhand smoke that lingers on coworkers' clothing and furniture can easily trigger a migraine. Keep abortive medications close at hand, and ensure that adequate drinking water and healthy snacks are available.

 Question

How can I explain my needs to my boss and coworkers?
If necessary, obtain a doctor's letter documenting your migraine and treatment plan and present it to your employer. Use physicians as a resource; they will have suggestions on the best way to manage migraines in the workplace.

Line of Work

If migraines strike fast, hard, and often, career choices may be affected. Some positions require specified working hours every day, and failure to appear (especially on an irregular basis) can be grounds for dismissal. Consider the degree of structure required by a potential place of employment before applying for a job. Employment with flextime and telecommuting may be a good choice for the migraineur who frequently requires an adjusted working schedule.

In some cases, those prone to chronic and severe migraine cannot maintain steady employment. If there appear to be no job prospects due to the amount of time missed for migraine-related illness, filing for SSDI (Social Security Disability Insurance) coverage and SSI (Supplemental Security Income) may be the last recourse. Remember that employers have a duty to provide reasonable accommodations for disability, but it may or may not be reasonable to provide a work schedule that changes on a weekly basis. Other possibilities include short-term medical leave under the federal Family and Medical Leave Act. Proving that a migraine sufferer is a qualified individual for Americans with Disabilities Act (ADA) coverage can be tricky, so contacting an employment or disabilities attorney may be required.

Seasonal Strategies

One of the more frustrating aspects of migraine treatment is the unpredictability with which migraines tend to strike. Eliminating triggers and keeping an accurate headache diary are two of the most helpful things a patient can do, along with supportive medical treatment, but some days it seems as if migraines attack for no apparent reason. They can be as irregular as the weather!

What does the weather have to do with migraines? As it turns out, seasonal variations in temperature, brightness, humidity, and a host of other factors can be a very good clue into migraine patterns. In a study conducted in Norway, researchers conducted a survey of 169 female migraineurs. Norway is located on the edge of the Norwegian Sea, and straddles the Arctic Circle. Because of its extreme north location on the globe, Norway experiences brighter than usual sunlight during the summer months and the "midnight sun" phenomenon, where the sun is visible twenty-four hours a day in midsummer. The study concluded that a significant percentage of migraineurs suffered attacks due to overexposure to sunlight and that the amount of exposure to light was a contributing factor to the number and intensity of migraines experienced.

 Fact

Bright lights are a well-known migraine trigger, and sunshine also has the potential to worsen an existing migraine. Wearing sunglasses or a wide-brimmed hat or limiting visual exposure to sunlight are appropriate strategies for migraine prevention.

Most research shows consistent results when it comes to the effects of weather, humidity, and air pressure on migraines. In a 1999 study conducted by the Robbins Headache Clinic in Illinois, it was shown that 47 percent of female migraine sufferers (and 34 percent of men) felt that changes in weather precipitated a migraine. Forty percent of women (and 31 percent of men) noted sunlight as a migraine trigger as well.

Watch the Barometer

Many migraineurs note seasonal variations in migraines—more headaches tend to appear during the fall and spring seasons. It is generally thought that changes in air pressure are to blame for the increased prevalence of migraine attacks during specific seasons. Rigorous reading of a barometer can help predict when seasonal migraines may occur and can give the migraineur additional preparation for a possible attack.

Sudden changes in air pressure appear to trigger migraines in many individuals. Average air pressure at sea level is 29.92 inches. When reading a barometer on a "typical" day near sea level, the needle (or digital display) will read around 29.9. On cloudy days that signal rain (often encountered in the fall), barometric pressure drops. Conversely, on clear and calm spring days, barometric pressure rises. While you cannot change the weather, you can change your routine and medication to account for variations in air pressure.

Note that no specific weather (sunny or cold, rainy or snowy) appears to have a consistent effect on migraine patterns. According to research conducted at the New England Center for Headache, it is the change in temperature, humidity, and air pressure that seems to trigger an attack. For example, a rainy day (with little sunshine) that is followed by a bright day (with many hours of bright sunlight) can provoke an attack. This insight can be used preventatively, allowing migraineurs to carry medications following weather conditions that are potential triggers. The preventative medications can then be taken at the first warning sign of a migraine.

Allergies

Seasonal allergies are another potential migraine trigger. When pollen fills the air, those who are sensitive to it suffer from inflamed sinus passages. If allowed to fester, this condition can easily lead to a sinus headache, characterized by pain and pressure in the face and upper jaw. The inflammation, called sinusitis, thus causes a sinus headache that can, in some cases, trigger a migraine.

Avoid getting to the point where pollen and blooming vegetation cause a sinus headache. If itchy and watery eyes, sneezing, and a stuffy nose accompany the arrival of spring, work with an allergist to determine the sources of your allergies and the most effective treatment. Daily medication, nasal sprays, sinus rinses, and allergy shots are all possible ways to control allergy sensitivity and lessen the likelihood of an allergy attack. Managing allergies can help prevent sinus headaches, which can in turn help avoid a migraine trigger. In some cases, the variation in pollen and general allergen level is what triggers a migraine directly (which can be confused with a sinus headache). Controlling allergies may help in either case.

Travel

While many people benefit from a change in routine, or anything that breaks up the tedium or monotony of their everyday lives, such change can be a migraine trigger to those who are particularly sensitive to disruptions in routine. The act of traveling is probably not to blame as much as it is the change in environment. Travel usually brings with it a change in weather, sleep, and diet.

Sometimes, though, the travel itself could contribute to the triggering effect. Migraineurs tend to be more sensitive than the general population to motion sickness. Long car rides, any sort of travel by sea, or even air travel lends itself readily to motion sickness because the body is changing acceleration and direction without the brain's foresight into these changes. Altitude is also a trigger factor for some people. See Chapter 6 for more information about how to mitigate and work around these potential triggers.

Happy Trails

How can migraineurs manage a migraine-free vacation? Being prepared goes a long way toward having a successful trip. If a certain breakfast cereal is an important part of your routine, for example, bring it with you. Try to go to bed and rise at the same times that you normally do, since maintaining predictable sleep patterns will help ward off a migraine attack. If you know that you cannot get comfortable sleeping on a hotel pillow, bring your own pillow from home. The extra luggage is well worth it when the alternative is missing part of a vacation due to migraine.

Travel Phobia

For migraine sufferers, getting migraines under control (or at least to the point where you know what your triggers are) is a major life accomplishment. It can take years to recognize these triggers, and doing so involves painful trial and error. When you finally feel in control of your migraines, it is as if an enormous weight has been lifted.

⊏ Essential

Make sure to bring both abortive and preventative medication in your carry-on baggage on any trip. Pay attention to early warning signs of an impending migraine and address those symptoms promptly. Educate travel partners about migraines so that friends and family can help with trigger avoidance.

Travel has the potential to upset this precious balance. New foods, surroundings, weather, and smells can wreak havoc with anyone who is susceptible to headaches, and even more so to the migraineur. Avoiding travel at all costs is possible, but it puts rather harsh limitations on the ability to visit friends and family, not to mention travel that might be required for work.

If a decision has been made to travel, prepare as much as possible. Talk to a physician about medications specific for travel-related anxiety. Always bring regular medication, and try to mitigate changes to routine as much as possible. However, in some cases, that weekend trip to the Poconos or that already-stressful family reunion might be worth skipping. If the trip in question is really unnecessary or not wanted in the first place, give it a miss.

Inspiration: Famous Migraineurs

If you suffer from migraine, take solace in the fact that you are not alone. In fact, you are in rather good company! Many famous individuals throughout time have had migraine headaches, and it did not dampen their ability to make significant contributions to history.

Artists and Writers

Vincent Van Gogh (1853–1890) was best known for his signature Dutch impressionist style, but he was also a migraineur. So was Claude Monet (1840–1926), a French impressionist best known for works such as *On the Bank of the Seine.*

Virginia Woolf (1882–1941) was an English novelist who is generally considered to be one of the founders of modern literature. She produced such titles as *Mrs. Dalloway* and *To the Lighthouse* while suffering from frequent migraines. Her erratic behavior was, at the time, attributed to depression and nervous breakdowns, but scholars today think migraine disease was a more likely culprit.

Some neurologists and medical historians also believe that the Reverend Charles Lutwidge Dodgson, better known as Lewis Carroll (1832–1898), experienced migraine with aura. Carroll does describe chronic vascular head pain in his personal letters, and researchers believe his hallucinogenic descriptions in *Alice in Wonderland* are an indication that he had firsthand knowledge of aura.

Many film and television stars also suffer from migraine; a short list includes Elizabeth Taylor, James Cromwell, Marcia Cross, and Whoopi Goldberg. Despite living very public lives, many actors, actresses, singers, and other performers have found techniques for managing their migraines.

Politicians and Athletes

Throughout time, many famous politicians have also suffered from migraines. Thomas Jefferson (1743–1826), the author of the Declaration of Independence and primary force behind the Louisiana Purchase, was thought to have experienced migraines throughout his life. Leaders from Julius Caesar (100 B.C.E.–44 B.C.E.) to Ulysses S. Grant (1822–1885) were also reportedly migraineurs.

Those who use their bodies as skillfully as their minds are not exempt from the pain of migraine either.

Professional athletes who live with migraine disease include NFL players Zach Thomas and Terrell Davis. Pro-Bowler Davis started the Terrell Davis Migraine Foundation in 1998 to raise awareness of the condition. The NBA has also been home to several migraineurs, including Scottie Pippen, Steve Francis, and Jason Kidd. And baseball pros Johnny Damon, Angel Berroa, Joe Girardi, and Jonathan Papelbon deal with migraines on the diamond and in the outfield. Professional athletes who are also migraineurs excel in just about every other playing field, including golf (Fred Couples and Kathryn Marshall), track (Gail Devers), and hockey (Pat LaFontaine and Henrik Lundqvist).

Migraine does not discriminate. It affects individuals from all walks of life, professions, and cultures. What sets migraineurs apart is not who they are or what they do, but how they take control of their lives and their disease.

CHAPTER 15

Family and Friends

ONE OF THE biggest challenges of living with migraines is educating the people around you about the true nature and impact of the condition. The people who form our support networks, family, and friends, are the backbone of our emotional well-being. Migraineurs, more than most people, must rely on the understanding and empathy of those they are close to, for both emotional and physical support. How can these people be helped in their understanding of migraines?

Not "Just a Headache"

For many people who have never had a migraine episode, or any severe headache, migraines can sound like a bad headache. Sufferers know this to be false, but the general perception among the uninitiated is that migraines are no big deal. How do you convince the people you live and work with that migraine is a serious problem?

Explanation

Start by pointing out that migraine is fundamentally different from other types of headaches. Refer to the table on the next page to see some of the most significant differences.

Migraines Versus Normal Headaches

Migraine	Normal Headache
Requires specialized abortive and preventative medications	Dissipates on its own with over-the-counter pain analgesics
Can last up to seventy-two hours	Generally lasts no more than a day
Usually requires bed rest and removal from external stimuli	Can be worked through
Can be accompanied by aura and visual disturbances	No aura
Sensitivity to lights, sounds, smells	Sensitivity to sounds
Comes with nausea and vomiting	No gastrointestinal upset
Features a prodrome and post-drome headache phase	Is a single headache event

Sharing

Free and open discussion is crucial to educating people as to the true nature of a migraine episode. Be patient and take the time to explain why a migraine is not "just a headache." Efforts spent on education in the beginning can be rewarded with empathy and compassion later.

If one's own personal knowledge of the subject proves insufficiently convincing, supply more professional sources. Share books, magazine articles, and research studies with friends and family. Bring your spouse or significant other to your next doctor's appointment so he can hear firsthand about your treatment plan and side effects of medications. To the extent that they are willing and able, actively engage your support system in your migraine management.

Educating Family and Friends

Of the world's population, only a small percentage (around 5 percent) manage to live completely headache free. That is an astounding number, but it means that head pain is something nearly everyone can relate to. Use this to your advantage when discussing migraines with close friends, and try to provide a frame of reference or an example. "A migraine is like being at a rock concert, standing inside one of those giant speakers, while having the stomach flu."

Allow others to help you by making your recovery needs (e.g., a dark and quiet room) clear to all. Show other adults in the household where you keep your migraine medications and any other needed supplies in the event that you are unable to retrieve them. But be sure to launch your education efforts when you're feeling well, not when you are in the middle of a migraine episode.

Familial Tendencies

Remember that migraines tend to run in families. The exact nature of how migraine might be inherited is still largely unknown, but it is well documented that having parents or other close relatives with migraines increases your own predisposition to having them.

Fact

Thirty-six million Americans are affected by the pain and stigma of migraine. That number has increased dramatically in recent years, due to more accurate diagnoses and heightened awareness. In any given year, close to 90 percent of people will have at least one headache, and more than 300 million people around the world will suffer a migraine.

What this means is that if you suffer from migraines, the odds are in your favor that someone else in your family does too. Where possible, do some research and try to locate these individuals; act as a mutual support system for each other. Take advantage of their knowledge of family dynamics to improve your own relationships with family members who cannot understand the extent of migraine disease.

Hidden Sufferers

It's also possible that some of those family members may not even realize that they have migraines. It is thought that close to 14 million people in the United States are undiagnosed migraineurs. The migraine sufferer is in a particularly beneficial position when it comes to recognizing the same suffering in people around him or her. Share your knowledge, and encourage anyone experiencing "the worst headache of their life" to consult a physician as soon as possible.

Peer Support Groups

Sometimes the only way to get adequate support for living with migraines is from fellow migraineurs. Friends and family mean well, and coworkers can empathize to the best of their abilities. However, there are times when you just need to talk to someone who has stood in your shoes, and who can share insights, compassion, heartaches, and humor.

When Peer Support Is Required

Migraines take their toll on the migraineur, to be sure, but they can also be draining for your support network. Constant reliance on family members for emergency child care, for example, may use up their goodwill when it comes to "optional" outings such as an evening work meeting or a movie with a friend. If a spouse is spending an inordinate amount of time cleaning the house or driving to doctor's appointments, she will eventually start to burn out. Protect the ones you love by letting them know how much you value their support, but also develop a network of outside help for chores and child care (paid or otherwise), and seek out and take advantage of peer support.

E-Mail Lists

A convenient way of receiving online support for migraines is from e-mail lists, sometimes called listservs. These lists work by subscription; generally someone has to be accepted to the list by a moderator, and that approval allows them to send and receive messages. Because the audience is so diverse, e-mail list queries usually get responses back within a few hours. Also, most lists allow subscribers to receive either individual messages, or a once-a-day digest with the day's messages compiled into a single e-mail.

If you don't enjoy web browsing and don't need an immediate response, e-mail lists are a terrific choice. Lists exist for general migraine sufferers, and there are others specifically for triggers, treatments, surgeries, and other aspects of migraine management. On the other hand, try not to let migraine or fear of migraine take over your life. Remember, when you are feeling well, the focus needs to be on wellness and enjoying life.

Essential

New e-mail lists are always being created, so there is good variety. The only things required to take advantage of e-mail lists are a computer with Internet access, and an e-mail program. If you don't find a list that meets your needs, it is easy to start your own. See Appendix A in the back of this book for more online resources.

Chats and Boards

One of the fastest ways to get quick feedback from fellow migraine sufferers is by reading and posting in an online forum. Pick the means that works best for you: chat rooms offer immediate feedback from whoever else happens to be online, whereas bulletin boards let you look through all the questions and answers that others have posted recently. If you are fast-paced and want to "talk" (or type) to another person in real time, go with a chat. If you prefer to peruse a series of questions and read all the answers that others have provided, boards may be the best choice.

 Question

What are some of the best online boards for asking migraine questions?

My Migraine Connection:
http://forums.healthcentral.com/discussion/migraine/forums

Worldwide Migraine Meetup:
http://migraine.meetup.com/boards

Revolution Health:
http://www.revolutionhealth.com/forums/headache/migraine

Online Medical Questions

There is a wide range of online options when it comes to technical migraine support. Many medical Web sites offer "Ask a Physician" pages, where you can e-mail questions and receive answers back in a short amount of time. Most of these sites retain your anonymity while providing you with another point of view to supplement that of your regular team of physicians. Providing as much information as possible will allow the doctors to better assess your situation and give you a more thorough answer to your query.

Remember, though, that asking questions online is no substitute for speaking to your own physician. Online question-and-answer sessions are a terrific way to validate new treatments or get suggestions for your existing treatment plan, but never rely on them exclusively.

Appendix A has a list of Internet resources for online migraine support.

Meeting in Person

For those who do not spend a lot of time online, or are uncomfortable seeking support from virtual strangers, consider one of the multitudes of "real world" support groups. The National Migraine Association and the National Headache Foundation both maintain a list of support groups organized by state. Similarly, the American Council for Headache Education is a good starting point to finding a group in your city.

Another good place to look for support groups is at a local hospital or medical center. All groups need some place to meet, and many of them use hospital meeting rooms after hours. Talk to your physician or call the hospital's community outreach department to inquire about migraine support groups in your area.

Sanity Strategies for Parents

Parenting is a full-time, year-round job. Unfortunately, migraine management can sometimes feel like a full-time job as well. Parents with migraines need to learn ways of controlling their medication, treatment, and triggers without the children feeling like their parent is absent.

When migraines first become a serious and chronic health issue for a parent, emotions abound. When it comes to parenting, unfortunately, one of the predominant emotions may be guilt. Migraineurs inevitably have less time to spend with their children, and some of their "free" time may be spent at doctor's offices, researching treatments, trying new medications, and riding the emotional roller coaster that often accompanies a diagnosis of migraine.

The Emotional Toll

Migraine can affect personality to the extent that the migraineur has a new understanding of pain. Migraine sufferers are intimately familiar with head pain; even when migraines are controlled with medication and trigger avoidance, the intensity of migraine pain is unforgettable. Sufferers have a special understanding of pain and, as a result, can be more tolerant of (and sensitive to) pain in others.

On the other hand, constantly having to confront pain can take a toll on one's emotional well-being. Migraineurs may feel exhausted and spent after an episode, but they can also become cranky and short-tempered in the early throes of an impending attack. This variability in how parents present themselves can be confusing and hurtful to their children.

Consistency, as much as possible, is a workable strategy. Children should be taught about the myriad emotions that accompany migraines, but parents should also strive to present a consistent front. When you can no longer keep up a pleasant face around the children, or when you feel that your children are becoming frightened by your behavior, call someone from your support network to take care of them. Children are resilient and can handle an amazing number of different situations, and it is beneficial for kids to learn how their parents manage their disease. However, if you are starting to feel guilty about the way you sometimes behave around them, remove yourself from the equation until the migraine abates.

Child Care and School Functions

When a migraine attack begins, the last thing someone wants to worry about is who will take care of the kids. Plan ahead by pre-arranging emergency child care with friends, relatives, or a drop-in daycare center. Make arrangements for someone to pick the children up from school if a daytime migraine leaves you completely incapacitated and unable to drive.

Having these plans in place will contribute to your peace of mind, in addition to making the children feel secure and comfortable. Children easily pick up on parental anxiety, and especially when Mom or Dad can't take care of them for a few hours, it will be very reassuring for the kids to understand that there is a backup plan in place. Along those same lines, arranging overnight care for the children is an extra step that should be taken by single parents, especially migraineurs with very young children.

Migraines do not always have the best timing, and may occur when a parent is scheduled to lead a field trip, give a talk in a child's classroom, or drive the morning carpool. As with the treatment of a migraine itself, prevention is one of the best solutions. Give your children's school all the relevant information they might need, including alternate contact numbers for people who can pick up your children from school. Always carry a cell phone, especially if you are leading a field trip or are responsible for someone else's children, so that you can contact an emergency backup person should it become necessary.

 Question

How much do I need to tell other parents about my migraine disease?
Where other parents are concerned, there is no need for full migraine disclosure. Rather, inform other parents as needed. Make it known that you might occasionally have to ask for another parent to take your place, for example, and arrange for a familiar parent to take your children home with her in an emergency

Timing

Migraine management should be planned, insofar as planning for the unpredictable is possible. Some migraine triggers occur at fairly predictable times, and parents can plan care for their children around those specific times. Menstrual migraines, for example, tend to occur around the same time every month. Use that knowledge to help prepare your children for the possibility that Mom might be out of commission for a few hours.

But make sure that children understand, to the best of their abilities, what is going on. The more they understand about the disease, the better equipped they will be to deal with the consequences.

When menses approaches and migraine symptoms begin, let the children know that they may be heading to Grandma's for the night. Special bonding can take place while you are helping them pack a bag, telling them a story, and giving extra hugs.

Genetics and Support

If you suffer from migraines, there is a good chance that at least one, if not all, of your children will encounter migraines as well. As an adult with experience in migraines, though, you are well situated to help children adjust and adapt. Pass on the benefits of your experience, and treat all migraine signs and symptoms seriously. Never assume that a child is "too young" or "too healthy" to fall prey to migraines, as they can strike any child at any age.

Essential

If your child is having difficulty coping with your migraine disease, consider an appointment with a counselor or child therapist. This will allow her to discuss her feelings without fear of hurting yours. Talk to your child's pediatrician about options near you. You can also inquire about children's support groups that may be appropriate.

Whether or not your child experiences migraines, she will still be affected by your migraine disease. While parents can offer assurances and be the primary source of information for their children, sometimes kids simply need to talk to other kids. Talk to your physician or local hospital about support groups for children who have parents living with chronic diseases. This kind of environment can help children feel less alone and will have peers with whom they can discuss the trials and tribulations of parental illness. This extra outlet for their thoughts and feelings will also relieve pressure from Mom and Dad, who may take on full responsibility for the impact of their migraines on their children. Engaging in an external support network is a win-win situation for parents and children alike.

Putting Yourself First

Moms and dads are superheroes. The adventures of Superman and Wonder Woman pale in comparison to the tasks that parents accomplish every single day. Getting everyone dressed, fed, and sent to school is only the tip of the iceberg. Working parents have to keep the house clean, maintain the yard, work a full day, pick up the kids, attend to homework, and get the kids fed, changed, and happily secure in their beds. "Me time? No way!" say many parents; by the time the children and work have been attended to, the day is simply over. Add migraine management into the equation, and parental achievement becomes magnified even further.

Taking the Time

Parenting and migraine experts agree that breaks are necessary. Parenting is exhausting. Managing migraines is exhausting. The pain of a migraine attack is exhausting. With all these multiple sources of exhaustion, how do migraineurs make time for themselves?

Making time for oneself requires commitment—as much commitment as, say, it takes to bring a child to soccer practice for a full season. Reinforce to family members that you need time just for you, and that that time is to be taken seriously. If necessary, schedule appointments with yourself on the family calendar! Expect your family to honor your time alone, and then be sure that you actually take it.

What to do with your newfound freedom? Many migraineurs enjoy simple time alone to reflect on their current pain-free day and enjoy the moment. Building a conscious appreciation of healthy periods gives you something to look forward to later and allows you to get through a migraine with the understanding that this, too, shall pass, and pain-free periods of time will follow.

Essential

If relaxing doesn't appeal to you, use the time to do things that you might not be able to when suffering an attack. Write letters, run errands, get caught up on bill paying, and do any other mundane tasks that let you feel more caught up with the rest of your life.

Realizing Your Worth

Many migraineurs have a low sense of self-esteem. The constant threat of an attack, as well as the social stigma of a chronic disease, can contribute to feelings of shame and worthlessness. The worse you feel about yourself, the less likely you are to value yourself enough to demand a break.

Defuse this cycle by understanding that migraines are not your fault, and there is no blame to be placed. Self-worth is derived from strength of character, values, morality, and the totality of a person's being. It is not diminished by disease. Take time for yourself because, in four easy words, you are worth it!

State of Mind

Happiness rubs off on those around us. When we are in a good mood, smiling, cheerful, and well rested, we project those emotions onto the people with whom we come into contact. Migraineurs may need to go to extra effort to achieve a rested, happy state, but arriving at that state benefits more than just themselves.

When migraine pain has abated and the postdrome has faded, rest and simple bliss can slowly make their way back. Irritability is a thing of the past. For some, the aftermath of a postdrome can feel euphoric, or it can feel like a hangover; eventually, though, normalcy resumes. After a painful migraine, normalcy seems twice as good as it did before.

When They Just Don't "Get It"

Even among loved ones, migraines remain a source of contention. Why does the migraineur get so much "special treatment" from work and family? Why does Mom get to sleep in all day? The more pertinent question may be, why is it so difficult when friends and family don't seem to understand the pain involved with migraines?

Expectations

Part of the conflict stems from expectations. Loved ones, the people we surround ourselves with every day, are generally held to a higher moral standard than coworkers or casual acquaintances. Migraineurs expect them to understand all the issues surrounding the management of a chronic disease, and so they are disappointed when family fails to come through.

This disappointment is unfortunately a side effect of the human condition. People expect more from those they love. When you are failed by family and friends, it hurts because you did not anticipate their failure. Is the answer that migraineurs must lower the expectations they hold for their loved ones? A more practical solution lies in education. If friends and family are taught the true nature, experience, and ramifications of suffering migraines, they will have the tools to display both sympathy and empathy for the disease.

However, in some cases, despite your best efforts to educate, family and friends may not provide the support you need. When this happens, don't go it alone. Seek out help in migraine support groups or private counseling.

Totality

Remember that, despite the gravity and inconvenience of migraine disease, migraine suffers are more than their disease. They are mothers, doctors, friends, lawyers, and waitresses. Migraine disease does not define the individual. Rather, it becomes a part of one's identity. A large part, to be sure, but it is only a piece. True friends will be able to see beyond the migraine and support the individual behind the pain.

Fact

Perhaps you've heard the old saying that it takes more muscle power to frown than it does to smile. Fact or fiction, the reality is that smiling is free. Take advantage of this renewable source of goodwill to forgive those who simply "don't get it," and move on.

When dealing with those who are short-sighted, though, do not forget to smile. The simple act of smiling promises to brighten your day, relieve anxiety, and promote good feelings in those around you. At the end of the day, if someone does not want to understand the nature of migraines, no amount of explanation on your part will do the trick.

CHAPTER 16

Your Emotional Health

WHEN IT COMES to healing, the connection between body, mind, and spirit is well established. The human mind has an incredible ability to heal and relieve pain. It also has the capability to cause physical distress by succumbing to stress, fatigue, and negative energy. Disease is battled by both the body and mind, and maintaining your emotional health relies on the ability to successfully manage stress while simultaneously seeking empowerment.

Coming to Grips with a Chronic Disease

Chronic diseases, or diseases that are both recurring and long-lasting, are the single largest cause of disability and death in America. A "chronic" disease is one that is persistent, as opposed to a "recurring" disease that generally features periods of illness, alternating with periods of remission. Chronic diseases become a part of everyday life.

Recognition

One of the first steps toward understanding chronic disease is recognizing its existence. When did a simple headache turn into a chronic illness, many early migraineurs ask themselves? The fact is, migraine disease is considered a chronic illness, and has been since the nature of this neurological disorder became better understood.

Depression

It isn't unusual for depression to occur in people with chronic health conditions like migraine. The realization that migraines may be with you for the rest of your life can be overwhelming. And depression may not always appear at diagnosis; long-term management of a chronic health condition can leave you burnt out, and if you're having difficulty finding a treatment regimen that works for you, frustration and discouragement may set in. These issues can set the stage for depression.

Symptoms of depression are not always easy to recognize. If someone is feeling sad or anxious most of the time, appears to have lost interest in activities that they used to enjoy, has less energy and appetite than usual, or has trouble sleeping, the chances are good that they are experiencing depression. And depression among chronic disease patients is not unusual. Some studies show that between 30 percent and 60 percent of all patients diagnosed with a chronic illness report having feelings of depression and anxiety.

 Fact

Some of the symptoms of depression appear contradictory in nature. For example, either unintended weight gain or loss can be a sign of depression, as can excessive sleep or insomnia. Talk to your health care professional if you experience any of these symptoms.

The first step down the road to recovering from depression is acknowledging that depression exists and seeking help. Talk to your doctor about your feelings; she can refer you to a mental health professional or, in some cases, prescribe treatment herself. Fortunately, there are many effective treatments available for depression, including medication, talk therapy, or a combination of the two. In some cases, minor lifestyle changes such as increasing exercise and practicing good sleep hygiene can also help alleviate feelings of depression. These have the added bonus of also being positive lifestyle changes for migraine prevention.

Coping Strategies

Learning how to successfully cope with migraines and migraine treatment can be one of the largest undertakings of a person's life. Bringing the disease under control is a primary goal, but bringing the entire treatment process under control is equally important.

General Coping Skills

Most forms of disease management focus around the idea of establishing a united approach to dealing with chronic symptoms, physical disability, and emotional well-being. Future plans need to be considered as well. As the course of chronic migraine disease changes, new medications might be instituted, and the patient has to adapt to this new regime. Psychological issues can develop at any time. Furthermore, interactions with health care personnel can be highly varied in their complexity, and a coherent plan for dealing with pharmacists, doctors, neurologists, and other specialists must be formed.

For some, the easiest way to cope with the stress of a chronic disease is to seek professional help. Counseling can provide incredible support to those who welcome it. The simple act of having someone to talk to, whose role is to listen, can relieve the burden considerably. Because chronic disease has so many different facets, it may be useful to work with someone experienced in both providing support, and with facilitating communication among the different parties.

Essential

There are many online programs designed for individuals who choose to self-manage their chronic illness. These programs rely on the patient's ability and desire to manage the disease, as well as communicate with medical and support staff as required.

On the other hand, some types of people prefer to manage their disease by themselves. Perhaps they had a negative experience with a therapist, for example, or perhaps they simply are more comfortable when in control of all aspects of their treatment. For these people, self-management can be a very effective means of coping with both their diagnosis and their disease. Oftentimes, a patient's spouse contributes to managing the disease so that the patient can retain control but still have a supportive person to aid with making important decisions.

In the News

When dealing with migraine treatment, it can be tremendously useful to stay on top of the latest developments. New medications, or new combinations or usages of existing medications, can make a world of difference for the migraineur. While physicians read medical journals and attend trade gatherings, they have many patients and cannot devote as much attention to your case as you can. Be proactive about researching treatments and proposing them to your physician.

When it seems that a limit has been reached with traditional therapies, one excellent way to cope with the stress of migraine treatment is to seek alternatives. Consider alternative treatment options such as biofeedback, acupuncture, and acupressure, and talk to specialists in those areas about how you might incorporate these sessions into your treatment plan.

Stress Management

Being diagnosed with a chronic disease is a definitive trigger for stress, which is a physiological response that is often characterized as the body's "fight or flight" mechanism. When we perceive a situation that is dangerous to our well-being, blood pressure and heart rate rise, adrenaline pumps, muscles tense up, and other changes take place to ensure that we have the strength to either "fight" for our lives in a dangerous situation or "flee" to safety.

For many migraineurs, stress is a Catch-22 situation; not only does the life disruption and physical discomfort associated with migraine elevate stress levels, but increased stress itself can trigger a migraine attack. Fortunately, there are many tips and tricks that can be used to help manage stress more effectively.

Good and Bad Stress

First, recognize that not all stress is bad stress. In certain cases, stress can be a motivator. Positive stress stems from competition, deadlines, and other time-sensitive tasks that require action. While not everyone appreciates positive stress, some thrive under it. Eliminating stress entirely is probably not a practical or realistic goal. However, learning to turn bad stress into good stress is something that applies to many aspects of life.

Essential

Never underestimate a good belly laugh. One of the quickest ways to reduce stress, and bring a lasting smile to your face, is by laughing. Call up a friend who shares your sense of humor. Read a book of jokes. Allow yourself the freedom to see the humor in life, and feel the stress physically float away.

You can take several steps, such as the following, to help get these tasks under control:

- **Realize stressors.** Just as migraine sufferers need to become aware of triggers for their migraines, they should also be cognizant of what factors in their pain management plan are causing stress.
- **Be realistic about change.** Some factors, like doctor's appointments and medications, cannot be adjusted on a whim. Other factors are more flexible. Find the stressful things that you *can* change and take steps to change them.

- **Alter your approach.** If your natural reaction to stress is to fly into an angry frenzy, take purposeful breaths until you are calm. If you tend to shut down and cease functioning, practice intentional relaxation techniques that allow you to continue your daily tasks.
- **Don't try to do it all.** Overbooked? Downsize your schedule. Make a short list of those regular commitments you must keep (making sure that at least one or two on the list are those you enjoy, as well), then graciously resign from the rest.

Exercise and Sleep

Exercise is one of the healthiest and most successful ways of reducing stress. It allows the pent-up energy that stress has produced to dissipate in a safe manner. When done regularly, exercise allows people to maintain more control over decisions in their lives through the simple act of physical exertion. After exercising, the body releases endorphins that are chemically similar to opiates. And, as a bonus, endorphins also act as a natural analgesic, or pain reliever. We feel good and, as a result, stress is relieved.

On the other side of the table, sleep hygiene, or routinely getting a healthy amount of sleep each night, is also an effective and necessary way of managing stress. Exhausted people do not tend to handle stress well, and most people who are chronically stressed also tend to be chronically tired. In addition, inadequate sleep or disrupted sleep patterns can also be a migraine trigger. Being well rested puts people in a better state of mind to handle stressful situations. Similarly, research shows that individuals who are stressed tend to sleep shorter hours, sleep more fitfully, and tend to wake up not feeling rested.

Are you sleep deprived? Sleep deprivation is defined as a lack of appropriate sleep, with "appropriate" being between five and ten hours per night, depending on individual needs. Insufficient sleep affects brain function, making it more difficult for individuals to accomplish even simple tasks. Studies suggest that between 10 and 30 percent of Americans are sleep deprived.

If this number includes you, potential solutions include setting aside adequate time for sleep and making sure that your sleeping room is cool, dark, and comfortable. Chapter 10 has more information on sleep and migraine.

Hobbies

When dealing with a chronic disease, it is easy to let managing your pain and treatment become a full-time job. Between work, family, and chronic disease, there seems to be little time left to engage in the activities that used to be enjoyable and fulfilling.

Make time for activities that are fun! Doing what we like reduces our stress levels and makes more difficult tasks seem manageable. Sign up for a pottery class, join a walking group, or simply enjoy a cup of coffee in a café. The more you can do for yourself, the more relaxed you will be when it comes to the challenges of illness.

Psychological Triggers

There will always be people who simply rub you the wrong way. Seeing such a person can bring back a flood of memories about your last meeting, including hurtful things you might have said to each other, and you are instantly reminded of all the reasons why that person is no longer on your guest lists. Similarly, places can evoke negative memories, as can objects or songs. Psychological triggers are anything that you see, read, hear, or even smell that triggers a particular reaction.

Can emotional events, such as anger or grief, trigger a migraine? Consider the physiological effect of emotion. Extreme psychological duress can cause stress, which in turn causes physical changes such as increased blood pressure and heart rate. While the emotion itself may not trigger a migraine, its physiological associations can serve as triggers.

Taking Time to Relax

Children have the right idea when it comes to relaxing. If you have ever watched toddlers, you have seen them engaging in a frenzied flurry of activity until the moment at which they no longer want to be engaged. At that point, they simply drop to the floor and rest. When they are refreshed, up they pop and off they go.

Toddlers have a very affirmative sense of self-worth; the entire world revolves around them! While becoming as self-centered as a child may not be the best course of action (and it will not win you any points at home), learn to acknowledge your own self-worth. The more value you place upon yourself, the more likely you are to take the time needed for relaxation. For people with low self-esteem and a low sense of self-worth, working with a professional therapist could be helpful.

Music to Your Ears

To your stress-relief tool chest, add another important tool: music. The right sorts of music can be both energizing and relaxing, and this combination is perfect for reducing stress. Let memory aid in the selection of relaxing music. Try to recall a vacation that was particularly enjoyable and relaxing, such as a trip to the beach. A CD of ocean waves might, in that case, allow you to relax and recall that time when you were calm and at peace. If a recent hike in the wilderness proved soothing, look for a CD with bird sounds or wind rustling.

Relaxation and Meditation

If you cannot commit to an hour for relaxation, can you find ten minutes? Progressive relaxation offers a quick, simple means to relax the body and mind. More importantly, it can be done anywhere, without the aid of expensive equipment. This technique involves a conscious awareness of each and every part of the body, in succession from head to toe. As each body part is visualized and focused upon, muscles relax and tension dissipates. Best of all, progressive relaxation is a technique that can be used at work, on a bus, or lying in bed at night.

Yoga is one of the most popular methods of combining exercise, stress relief, and relaxation. Yoga involves stretching, positioning, breathing, strength, stamina, and flexibility. Instructors teach different yoga positions that work different parts of the body, and these poses can be executed extremely slowly, or relatively quickly. Yoga is a flexible system that can easily be adapted to an individual's physical limitations, and it is ideal for migraineurs because it does not involve high-impact activities that can act as triggers. If time is a consideration, yoga is a perfect outlet for stress relief because it can do double duty as both exercise and as a relaxation technique. Watch a yoga program on television or, if time permits, join a yoga class.

Meditation is another stress-relieving activity that allows both the body and mind to relax. The idea behind meditation is that attention can be focused outside the body, onto an object or idea. Focused breathing and postures are two of the central elements of meditation. Many Eastern religions around the world use meditation as a way of achieving a higher spiritual connection, and most religions incorporate meditation into their practice in some capacity. Consider learning more about meditation by reading, attending workshops, or working with an expert.

Essential

If music is sufficiently soothing and played at a low enough volume, it can also be used as a sleep aid. Look for music with rhythmic, repeating elements. Some people prefer natural sounds such as ocean waves and wind, while others find the monotonic, repeating sounds of African drumming to be more soothing.

Being an Empowered Patient

There was a time, years ago, when the family physician took the time to treat each and every one of our ailments. Children of previous generations were cared for by a single pediatrician, one who knew them well enough to recite their medical problems without a chart in sight during a leisurely visit in the examining room.

Today, things are different, and medical care is often much more impersonal. If you're in a managed care plan, you may see a different practitioner every time you visit the doctor's office. And you'll rarely spend much more than fifteen minutes with your doctor. So it's important for patients with any type of serious illness, and particularly one like migraines, to find a way to work within the health care system to receive the care they need.

 Fact

Medical mistakes and prescribed drug interactions are at an all-time high. Medical errors in the United States alone result in between 40,000 and 90,000 deaths annually. While computerized systems are designed to look for drug interactions, it's a good idea to talk to both your doctor and your pharmacist when starting any new drug.

Acceptance

One of the most important aspects to managing chronic illness, and to becoming an empowered migraineur, is acceptance. Migraine, or any other chronic disease, disrupts life. Recognition of this painful but important fact is necessary before it is possible to change your situation.

Along with acceptance, recognize that anxiety, fear, and even anger are appropriate emotional reactions to a chronic diagnosis. Life changing events come with some emotional cost. However, just as you would manage the disease with a treatment plan, emotions can be channeled as well. Often with the help of a trained counselor, you can develop strategies for dealing with these emotions and reestablishing control.

It is important to remember that there is no blame, responsibility, or failure associated with being diagnosed with a chronic illness.

Patients may experience these emotions, and they are valid ones. However, with sufficient time to grieve the loss of your past pain-free life, as well as time to acknowledge the role that pain may play in your future life, healing and empowerment can begin.

Taking Responsibility

Each physician comes to the table with his own personal opinion and viewpoint. He may not be aware of research out of his immediate line of expertise, or he may disregard certain therapies as "new and untested," or "old and irrelevant." The responsible patient has a duty to inform herself of all the options, and present these to her physician for discussion and evaluation.

One caveat here—remember that your doctor is your partner in health care, so present your questions and comments on migraine therapy in a collaborative, not a combative, way. There is a tidal wave of health information currently available to consumers on the Internet. This has been a double-edged sword for the medical profession. On the one hand, patient education is always a positive thing; a person who takes the time to seek out information on her condition and teach herself is more likely to adhere to a treatment program. But on the other hand, physicians have to spend increasing amounts of time dispelling health hoaxes and migraine myths, sometimes to the disbelief of patients who think that because something was on the Internet (or in the newspaper, for that matter), it has to be right. Always seek out health information from credible sources and communicate your findings with your doctor in the spirit of partnership.

Essential

You always have the right to go and seek a second opinion if you don't believe that your physician is listening to or addressing your treatment needs. At the end of the day, you are the one who has to live with the treatment decisions.

Empowered patients must take responsibility for their treatment plan right down to the details of prescription medication. The Internet abounds with online pharmaceutical indexes. With these tools, patients can easily look up the medications they have been prescribed and check to ensure that they do not have negative interactions with one another. Should the pharmacy filling the prescription check for interactions? Of course, but the reality is that mistakes can happen. Taking responsibility for your care helps ensure that these mistakes, if they occur, don't become a health hazard.

 Fact

> It's always a good idea to take notes at your doctor's appointments. But if anxiety or poor penmanship prevent you from taking accurate notes, try using an audio recorder for the question and answer portion of your visit. Be sure to explain your strategy to your doctor at the beginning of the appointment.

Most new physicians begin an examination with a family history. Do you really remember if your cousin twice removed or great-grandmother suffered from migraines? Create a family medical history, put it in writing, and place it in a folder that you bring to doctor's appointments.

No one is at her best while in a doctor's office. Doctors make people nervous, hence the infamous "white coat syndrome" where people who have normal blood pressure tend to get high readings at the doctor's office. Nervous people do not do a great job of listening or paying attention. Bringing a tape recorder to doctor's visits can help make sure that the entire conversation is documented and also gives you something to look back on later, when you have questions about something the doctor might have said.

Playing the Mediator

These days, it is common for migraineurs to see a number of different physicians and health care professionals. If you have other comorbid (or coexisting) medical conditions, the treatment picture gets even more complex. Coordinating the paperwork, records, visit notes, and treatment plans is something that must be done, and who better to do it than the person with the most vested interest in the case?

Remember that collaboration is the best way to ensure success. Make sure that the various doctors on your team communicate with each other, and make sure to sign all the relevant release forms so that they can share records on your care. Get to know the office manager in each practice so you can find the most efficient way to get files, lab results, and other important information where it needs to go. Create a reference list of contact information for all your health care providers to include in your chart at each provider's office. If all players are aware of the treatments and suggestions of the others, mistakes will be significantly reduced and patient care will be improved.

CHAPTER 17

Headache-Free Diet

DIET IS ONE of the most important aspects of migraine treatment and may seem like the element over which migraineurs can have the most control. However, food and beverage triggers aren't always so easily identified, and hidden additives can make pinpointing problems tough. Knowledge of migraine-inducing foods and additives, coupled with a careful reading of ingredients, can help you establish what foods are migraine triggers for you and help you to eliminate them from your diet.

Avoiding Food Triggers

It makes perfect sense to say that if a certain food acts as a migraine trigger, that food should be avoided. Unfortunately, simply steering clear of triggers is harder than it sounds. They can be difficult to identify and even more difficult to isolate and remove from your diet.

But by following a careful process of food logging and systematic dietary isolation, and allowing your body appropriate time to adjust and react to the changes, your dietary detective work will pay off with a reduced frequency of migraine attacks.

Isolating Problem Foods

The first rule of dietary isolation is to take it slowly. Eliminating ten foods at once may prove successful, but it will be nearly impossible to determine which foods were the triggers and which were benign. Remove one potential trigger food from your diet at a time.

If migraines abate, you may have gotten lucky on the first try. In most cases, however, patience is needed for this long and sometimes tedious process.

For example, if you decide to try substituting the artificial sweetener you usually use to sweeten coffee and foods with regular sugar, leave the rest of your diet unchanged. If a migraine presents itself on the second day of this attempt, you may assume that the sweetener is not a major trigger. However, if this particular migraine is less intense than is typical for you, keep making the sugar substitution until you are convinced that either the artificial sweetener is a trigger for you, or that it has no impact on the frequency and duration of your migraines. At that point, it is safe to proceed with removing a second triggering food from your diet. This process of elimination will eventually identify food triggers.

 Alert

Going cold turkey on dietary caffeine can actually cause headache. If you think caffeine may be a migraine trigger, gradually reduce the amount of it in your diet rather that cutting it out completely all at once. Reducing coffee intake by a cup each week is a good way to start.

Remember that some potential triggers can be hidden ingredients in some of the other foods you regularly consume. Artificial sweeteners are a good example; many "sugar-free" and low-calorie foods use them in abundance. Careful label reading is important to ensure that you exclude the trigger from your diet completely during this process of elimination and testing.

Exclude Triggering Foods

One of the best ways to avoid eating or drinking something at home is to keep it out of the house. Once it becomes clear what your trigger foods are, stop purchasing them. If anyone else in the house usually does the grocery shopping, leave them a written reminder stating which foods are forbidden.

What if one of your major trigger foods ends up being a child's or spouse's favorite? Look for substitutes that are suitable for everyone in the household. Carob, for example, can frequently be substituted for chocolate in many recipes. If the mozzarella on pizza triggers your migraines, try substituting a rice or soy cheese.

Another strategy is to designate a kitchen cabinet or pantry shelf as a place to store foods that are off-limits to the migraineur, but that the rest of the family can still continue to enjoy. The same can go for a designated drawer or shelf in the refrigerator. This keeps all of your potential problem foods in one area that you can easily avoid, leaving the rest of your kitchen as a migraine-free zone.

Committing to Change

Dealing with food triggers will be challenging to migraineurs. However, it is an important step in migraine management and should be treated as medically necessary. Having a good attitude about upcoming dietary changes will help tremendously in aiding both the patient and family members to adapt quickly. Be open-minded to food substitutes—the up side is that you may make some pleasant new discoveries that you would otherwise never have experienced. And remember the greater good: eliminating migraine triggers gives you a very good chance of decreasing the incidence of migraine attacks and leading to a better quality of life overall.

One of the most difficult things for migraine sufferers, when it comes to dealing with food triggers, is accepting the fact that dietary changes are usually permanent. Once a food trigger has been identified and removed from the diet, it needs to be removed from the diet from that point forward. Occasionally, some people are able to slowly add back trigger foods, but more often, sensitivities to certain foods do not go away with time.

Once a food has been eliminated for some number of years, the migraineur may not even want to add it back. If you have not eaten bananas in ten years, for example, you will have probably lost the taste for them and do not crave them any longer. If you do decide to add trigger foods back into your diet, add them one at a time, in small measures, and be prepared for a possible resurgence in headache frequency or intensity.

Reading Labels/Recognizing Hidden Triggers

Food labels carry important information for migraineurs and nonmigraineurs alike and allow you to identify potential dietary concerns such as trans fats, genetically engineered corn, and stealth calories. For someone suffering from migraine, not reading labels carefully can be the difference between a pain-free day and one spent in misery.

Unfortunately, even a conscientious label reader can mistakenly ingest foods laced with migraine triggers. Some ingredients are labeled with scientific names, ones that might not be easily recognized as triggers. Other labels might omit trigger ingredients, or hide them under the guise of "added flavorings and seasonings."

When in doubt, contact the manufacturer. They should be able to detail exactly which flavorings, seasonings, and food colorings are used in their products. If for some reason they cannot share that information, it might be wise to avoid the items in question if you suspect them of triggering migraine attacks.

 Fact

Glutamate, an amino acid, is actually found naturally in several foods including grapes, spinach, some aged cheeses, mushrooms, and tomatoes. Monosodium glutamate is the chemically manufactured version of glutamate.

MSG (monosodium glutamate)

MSG is a food additive that is commonly used to enhance flavor. It is found in many different processed foods, including flavored potato chips and other snacks, sauces, soups, and prepared meals.

It is also present in many different types of restaurant food, the most notable being fast food and Asian cuisine.

Any time a food is considered "seasoned" or "flavored," read the ingredients carefully to check for MSG. For example, most plain potato chips, corn chips, and pretzels do not contain MSG. However, most flavored versions (barbeque, sour cream and onion, ranch, etc.) do contain MSG, unless the brand is "all natural" or explicitly says it does not use MSG.

MSG is created when protein is broken down and fermented; particular bacteria excrete glutamic acid that is then filtered and added to salt to create the substance known as MSG. MSG works by stimulating the taste buds into making food seem more appealing. Some studies have suggested that MSG might even appeal to an extra fifth fundamental taste, in addition to the typical ones of sweet, salty, sour, and bitter. Animal studies have also suggested that ingesting large amounts of food with MSG can lead to high blood sugar and obesity.

Among the foods and dietary substances known by researchers to potentially trigger migraines, MSG holds a prominent place on the list. Potential reasons for its triggering power include the fermentation inherent to the MSG-making process, and the possibility that MSG actually alters brain function by affecting the behavior of serotonin.

 Alert

Anyone familiar with migraine triggers should have picked up on two major red flags with the description of how MSG works. Fermented products, or ones based on the process of sugar being converted to alcohol by way of yeast, are well-known migraine triggers. Blood sugar changes can also trigger headaches and migraine attacks in many individuals.

Be aware that there are several different "flavor enhancers" that have similar properties to MSG and may act as triggers in much the same way. Some of the similar enhancers include:

- BHA or BHT
- Hydrolyzed vegetable protein (HVP) or hydrolyzed plant protein (HPT)
- Modified food starch
- Carageenan
- Maltodextran

A trial exclusion of these flavor enhancers from your diet can help you to determine if they are a trigger for you.

Color Additives

Sometimes the triggering agent can be in the coloring rather than the flavoring. FD&C yellow #5 (also called tartrazine dye) is a color additive that is found in soft drinks and candy. It can also be found in medications, so read all prescription and over-the-counter bottles carefully to be sure vitamins and other drugs do not contain it. Be aware that yellow dye is used in more than just yellow foods! Yellow is used to create other colors, including orange, green, blue, and maroon, so read food labels and ask the pharmacist about color additives before picking up any new medication.

 Question

Are FD&C color additives only found in food?
FD&C stands for food, drug, and cosmetics, and these additives can be found in all three types of products. The U.S. Food and Drug Administration (FDA) regulates the use of these color additives to ensure their overall safety for consumers.

Sugar and Sweeteners

It is normal to expect that when people eat sugar, their blood sugar levels rise. However, migraineurs tend to be more sensitive than most to changes in blood sugar. This rapid change may trigger migraine, but it can be avoided by limiting intake of refined sugars. Hypoglycemia, or low blood sugar, is a potential migraine trigger for children and adolescents in particular. There appears to be a correlation between low blood sugar and more intense migraine. Some migraineurs benefit from a small amount of sugary drink at the onset of a headache or migraine because it quickly raises the blood sugar. If sugar sensitivity seems to be a migraine trigger, consult a dietician or nutritionist to plan out a detailed meal schedule.

Artificial sweeteners can also be a culprit. Staying within one's ideal weight range contributes to overall fitness and well-being. For many people, reducing sweets and fatty foods is an integral part of a diet plan. Fried foods can be substituted with baked, and sweets are often traded for foods made with artificial sweeteners that have far fewer calories than sugar.

Aspartame

Aspartame is a chemical compound that consists of two different amino acids—aspartic acid and phenylalanine. It is sold as a sweetener, and is also used as an ingredient in numerous sugar-free, diet, and low-calorie foods and drinks.

Several studies have shown a link between aspartame and migraine. Aspartame appears to lower levels of serotonin in the body; this change in regulation can be enough to either trigger a migraine, or worsen an existing headache. Migraineurs who are sensitive to aspartame should avoid foods and beverages with Equal, Nutra-Sweet, Canderel, or any other sweeteners that list aspartame among their ingredients.

Other Artificial Sweeteners

There are many types of artificial sweeteners other than aspartame. Saccharine (Sweet 'n Low) is one of the oldest available sweeteners; and while it's been linked to health issues, migraine is not among them. Sucralose is a newer sweetener that is sold under the brand name Splenda and is found in many foods and beverages. While it is not a frequent trigger for migraine, there are several published case reports of migraine triggered by sucralose in the medical literature. If you notice a sensitivity to sucralose, place it on the elimination list and see if migraines are reduced in frequency or intensity.

Comfort Foods

As described in Chapter 6, one of the major culprits when it comes to food triggers is amines. These are substances derived from amino acids, which are molecules that help form the building blocks of life. Amines include several compounds (tyramine, phenylethylamine, and histamine) that are known migraine triggers.

Unfortunately, many typical "comfort foods" can contain these substances. Comfort foods are simple, hearty, and familiar; they often may be the foods that you grew up eating. The good news is that with careful substitutions, the foods you know and love can still be consumed without fear of triggering a migraine attack.

Chocolate

While clinical research findings have conflicted on whether a correlation between chocolate and migraine exists, many migraineurs consider it a primary trigger food. Chocolate contains phenylethylamine, and histamine, which have been linked to migraine.

Chocolate lovers are not doomed to a life without a hint of cocoa. Carob makes a decent substitute for chocolate. It is a member of the legume family and has several advantages over chocolate: it contains no caffeine and does not have the triggering phenylethylamine. It is also a nutritious food, containing protein and vitamins A, B, and D in addition to calcium, potassium, and magnesium. However, both carob and chocolate contain tannins, so if you have a sensitivity to this substance, carob may not be an effective substitute.

Meats and Barbeque

Hot dogs are an ultimate American food. Unfortunately, they are swimming in sodium nitrite. This is a chemical compound that acts as a food preservative and color fixative and is found in most cured meats, sausages, bacon, pepperoni, hot dogs, jerky, and commercially dried fish products. Sodium nitrate is added to processed meats in order to increase the shelf life and maintain color.

A craving for hot dogs might be satisfied by consuming another type of meat. Fresh beef, chicken, and pork do not contain sodium nitrate and are not thought to trigger migraines when prepared correctly. If the hot dog craving simply will not disappear, try substituting tofu hotdogs or other vegetarian sausages, or look for all-natural brands that do not contain artificial preservatives.

Hearty southern foods such as barbeque and fried chicken are synonymous with comfort food. However, they can be triggering foods, depending on the preparation. When fried chicken is prepared at home with known ingredients, consuming it can be a migraine-free experience. Fried chicken from most chain restaurants, though, tends to be loaded with MSG, a major migraine trigger.

When it comes to food cooked outdoors, be wary; it is possible to have an allergy to the smoking technique used to create that fantastic-tasting barbeque. Different types of wood are often used in barbeque, in addition to or instead of charcoal and gas; common barbequing woods include cedar, hickory, apple wood, and oak. Anyone with seasonal allergies, or with sensitivity to nicotine smoke, may well have an allergy to "barbeque smoke." Headache can result and, depending on the migraineur, a migraine could be triggered. If trial and error proves that migraine is provoked after being outside at a barbeque, try remaining indoors during the next one (or skip it altogether).

Soups and More

Soup is symbolic of hearth and home and can be the ultimate comfort food because it is easily digested and appeals to our senses even when we are ill. When soup is made with prepared bouillon, however, it can contain a potential migraine trigger. Many brands of bouillon contain MSG, so read the ingredients when using a prepackaged soup mix. By using either homemade broth or non-MSG soup mix, soup can be enjoyed by all.

Fact

> The smell of fresh yeast-risen bread, rolls, and cake is reminiscent of home and family for many. Unfortunately, brewer's yeast can be a potential migraine trigger. If yeast sensitivity appears to cause migraines, omit fresh-risen breads from the diet and replace with flatbread or crackers.

Macaroni and cheese is a very typical comfort food, probably because it's something many of us remember from childhood. Generally, macaroni does not contain ingredients that trigger migraine. Cheese, however, is another story. Many types of cheese contain tyramine, an amino acid that is a potential migraine trigger. Aged cheese such as Parmesan, Pecorino Romano, Asiago, and hard cheddar tend to have the highest concentration of tyramine, so those should be the first ones to eliminate from your diet.

It is possible to continue enjoying dishes such as macaroni and cheese, but avoid using aged or moldy cheeses. Processed cheeses, made from unfermented dairy products, are better options, as is a cheese made from tofu or rice. Make sure that any processed cheese products you use don't have MSG or other triggering substances on their ingredients list.

Eating Out

Dining out with friends, family, and coworkers is one of life's little pleasures, but it can turn into a nightmare for a migraineur with food triggers. Learn to ask the right questions and avoid an unpleasant restaurant experience.

When you make the inevitable trip to the mall food court, avoid anything that might be fried or seasoned using MSG. Be wary of hamburgers, hot dogs, seasoned French fries, Asian stands, Mongolian barbeques, or anything else that offers sauces without clear lists of ingredients. Even many salad dressings contain MSG. The safest (and healthiest and least expensive) bet is to bring food from home, or stick to salads sans dressing, vegetable plates, or "healthy" fare, where you can readily ascertain every ingredient.

Alert

Not all fast food restaurants use MSG in their food. Of those that do, some dishes may be MSG free. Most company Web sites list a menu with "nutritional information" that mentions whether each item has MSG or not. Even sauces, dressings, and side items that are considered "plain" or "regular" flavor may contain MSG.

As with mall food, the major migraine risk when eating in a restaurant is MSG or other additives hidden in dishes. Asian restaurants tend to use MSG more than some other types of cuisine; they also make heavy use of soy sauce, another potential trigger food. When dining at a traditional full-service Asian restaurant, asking the wait staff to omit MSG from your order should enable you to enjoy the meal. Also, as MSG sensitivity is becoming more commonplace, many restaurants have stopped using MSG altogether. When in doubt, ask.

Bear in mind that fast food restaurants receiving prepared ingredients from large distribution centers will probably not be able to prepare your meal without MSG. Asking the staff may prove fruitless, as they may not receive sufficient training to know exactly what goes into their hamburgers, French fries, or chicken nuggets. Peruse the corporate Web site or call their customer service department to ask specifically which items contain MSG, BHT, or other additives and preservatives.

Supermarket Tips

Knowing one's migraine triggers can make a trip to the grocery store easier. However, a few simple tricks can further reduce the likelihood of inadvertently purchasing items that may actually end up being new triggers.

Some migraineurs swear by a "whole food" diet. Foods in this regimen include whole wheat, brown rice, low-fat dairy, soy, fresh fruits and vegetables, and fish high in omega-3 fatty acids. None of these foods are known to trigger migraine, and a diet clear of fried foods and refined sugars comes with its own set of health benefits. Shopping the "perimeter" of the store—where meat, produce, dairy, and other fresh whole foods are usually located—for the bulk of your shopping is a good strategy for avoiding overly processed and potential trigger foods.

Dairy

While fresh milk, butter and cream are not known to trigger migraines, there is a potential correlation with outdated dairy products. Always check the date on the carton, and try to buy products that are at least a week away from their posted sell-by date.

Yogurt and sour cream, on the other hand, are fermented products that contain tyramine, and should be avoided as potential triggers. Aged cheeses may also contain tyramine.

Fruit and Veggies

While whole fresh fruits and veggies contain no MSG or other added triggering chemicals, some of them contain naturally occurring substances that can provoke an attack. Citrus fruits contain tyramine, so they frequently appear on lists of migraine trigger foods. Bananas contain both histamine and tyramine, also both potential migraine triggers. Avocado and spinach may be a problem for the same reason.

Always check the labels on fruit and vegetables that are dried or dehydrated or that are in juice form. These may contain added sulfites, another known migraine trigger.

Besides fruits and vegetables, there are other foods that naturally contain migraine-triggering substances. Phenylethylamine-containing foods include cheese, chocolate, citrus, cocoa, and red wine. When avoiding tyramine-containing foods, make sure to skip aged cheese, beer and ale, fava beans, nuts, olives, pickles, red wine, salted or cured meat, sauerkraut, sour cream, soy sauce, teriyaki sauce, and yogurt.

Essential

Some common histamine-containing foods are aged cheese, beer and ale, banana, citrus, eggplant, fish, pineapple, red wine, spinach, strawberry, tomato, and yeast.

Drinking Smart: Alcohol and Caffeine

Dehydration is a known migraine trigger, so adequate fluid intake is an important part of a healthy lifestyle for the migraineur. However, many beverages can contain substances that have the potential to set off a migraine attack. So keeping a diary of what you drink to search for possible triggers is just as important as tracking your food intake.

Water should be the mainstay drink of choice for most migraineurs— it's additive-free, inexpensive, and noncaloric. You may be able to enjoy a variety of other beverages, but be aware of the additives and natural chemicals in many popular drinks so you can identify those that aren't compatible with your personal migraine management.

Alcohol

Not all alcoholic beverages are equal, and some may contain additional substances that can have an impact on migraine disease. Red wines, for example, are reported as a common trigger for many migraineurs, although studies have failed to reveal a connection between the two. For other people, beer or spirits may cause migraines.

Fermented drinks, such as red and white wines and beer, may contain histamine. Studies conducted by the National Institutes of Health show that histamine can induce migraine, either immediately or following a short delay. Many alcoholic drinks may contain tyramine in addition to histamine. A short list of drinks with tyramine includes red wine, beer, and champagne.

Up to 30 percent of migraine sufferers report sensitivity to beer, so eliminating it entirely would be a good way to determine whether it serves as a trigger. Distilled spirits, such as vodka, are not a common or well-known migraine trigger, but each migraineur is different. Experiment with one drink at a time, and keep a careful headache diary to help determine which drinks act as triggers.

Alert

Red wine contains tannins, which have been suspected to cause headaches. Tannin is a naturally occurring chemical that is present in grape skins, and it gives wine its dryness and bitterness. Since the process of red wine making includes the grape skins for color, it contains more tannin than white wine.

Caffeine

The most common drug in the United States, caffeine is one of the double-edged swords of migraine management. It is also prevalent in many over-the-counter migraine medications because it can be useful in stopping a migraine headache in its early phases. Caffeine acts as a vasoconstrictor and cardiac stimulant and, when taken in a small amount at the start of a migraine, can relieve headache pain. However, if caffeine intake is excessive, rebound headaches can become common when caffeine intake is withdrawn.

A possible solution regarding caffeine for migraineurs is to save it for emergencies. Enjoy decaffeinated coffee in the morning and use caffeinated soft drinks or coffee only when necessary to curtail a migraine attack. The caffeine will be more effective, and removing it largely from one's diet may reduce the number of headaches triggered by caffeine.

CHAPTER 18

Advocacy and Your Rights

BEYOND THE HEALTH and family challenges of living with migraines, this condition also brings with it a variety of legal and financial obstacles. Severe and unpredictable migraine may hamper your ability to hold a full-time job and require that you apply for some level of disability benefits. Or, you may face discrimination in the workplace from those who don't understand the condition, threatening your job security. The potentially high cost of migraine care can also place a strain on your economic well-being. Know what your insurance options and rights are, and what other public and private programs are available to bridge the financial gap.

Disability

The pain of migraine is not solely physical. Studies show that people suffering from the most severe migraines tend to also suffer financially and socially. It is estimated that close to 10 percent of migraineurs are unemployed; that is nearly twice the unemployment rate in the nation as a whole. When working becomes impossible, or discrimination interferes with the ability to keep a job, it may be necessary to consider applying for disability benefits.

The information below is intended to provide a wider frame of reference for the options that may be available to you, but it will be necessary to coordinate these resources with your medical team. Your health care provider's office can often help guide you through the potential maze of paperwork and regulations surrounding disability benefits, but you may also need to consultant an attorney specializing in disability law.

Definition

Does migraine disease qualify as a disability? The answer depends upon the degree to which a migraineur is able to continue a normal life. Generally speaking, to qualify as a disability, migraine disease must prevent an adult from being able to work for at least twelve months. That said, the law offers protection in a variety of forms for those suffering from a disability.

ADA Law

The Americans with Disabilities Act (ADA) serves to protect Americans with disabilities from discrimination under the law, including with regard to employment. ADA protection applies to individuals with a disability that "limits one or more major life activities." The language of the ADA is such that it can be construed to imply that individuals are protected not only for having a disability, but also for appearing to have a disability.

 Alert

Not sure if your migraine disease qualifies for disability benefits? Taking the Migraine Disability Assessment Questionnaire (MIDAS) may help you organize your options. This survey is available through The American Council for Headache Education and The National Migraine Association. It may also be administered in your doctor's office.

Title I of the ADA relates to employment. Any employer with fifteen or more employees is required to provide disabled people with equal opportunity employment, meaning they must be given the same opportunities as nondisabled people. Disabled people cannot be discriminated against when it comes to being hired or promoted, receiving bonuses, or participating in social functions. If such discrimination against an individual takes place, charges against the employer can be filed.

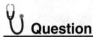
Question

Does migraine qualify as a disability under the ADA?
The answer generally must be derived from a careful study of the individual circumstances. One person may be able to continue working full-time despite the occasional migraine attack, for example, while another may be functionally disabled and unable to hold down a steady job.

To qualify for ADA protection, an individual must be considered "qualified." Can a migraine sufferer still perform the required functions of their job and, if so, can they do so consistently? Migraine pain rarely comes and goes on a schedule, so the question is a difficult one. Note also that all employers of more than fifteen people must provide "reasonable accommodation" for their employees. Is it reasonable to allow an employee to leave the office during a migraine attack? The answer probably depends on a number of factors, such as that person's role in the current project and whether another employee could replace her on a temporary basis, and the size and nature of the company or the specific department within the company. Other workplace accommodations might include replacing fluorescent bulbs in an employee's workspace or providing occasional breaks from the computer screen to reduce eyestrain.

Visit the ADA Web site for more information on protection in the workplace: *www.usdoj.gov/crt/ada*.

Social Security Disability
The Social Security Administration has two different programs under which disability money can be disbursed.

- Supplemental Security Income (SSI): This form of coverage is available to people who work and who have coverage under Social Security.
- Social Security Disability Insurance (SSDI): This form of coverage is available to people with low income and assets.

Start looking into the possibility of Social Security payments by calling the local Social Security office. You will be asked for documentation of your disease and other information, so plan to have the following at hand before making the call:

- All relevant medical records from hospitals, doctors, therapists
- Any and all records of medication and test results
- Your own employment history, including names, addresses, and job functions
- Your Social Security number

The Social Security Administration publishes a very informative booklet on how to apply for benefits. Obtain a copy and read it thoroughly.

Other Sources of Information

The 1973 Rehabilitation Act is a piece of United States legislation that provides rights and protections to individuals with disabilities. Section 504 of the Rehabilitation Act pertains largely to employment, stating: "No otherwise qualified individual with a disability in the United States, as defined in section 705(20) of this title, shall, solely by reason of her or his disability, be excluded from participating in, be denied the benefits of, or be subjected to discrimination under any program or activity receiving Federal financial assistance or under any program or activity conducted by an Executive agency or by the United States Postal Service."

Per this act, the implication for migraine sufferers working in a federally funded capacity is that if a migraine qualified as a disability, he or she could not be discriminated against. Accommodation plans must be developed in order to comply with the law. Charges can be filed against employers who refuse to supply a plan for such accommodation.

Additionally, many states offer disability protection under their laws. The California Fair Employment and Housing Act (FEHA), for example, protects Californians against unlawful harassment and discrimination in the general areas of both housing and employment. Employment discrimination is prohibited on the basis of race, color, religion, national origin, marital status, sex or sexual orientation, age, pregnancy, childbirth and, of interest here, physical or mental disability. The implication is that if an employer engages in discrimination against anyone with a verified disability, that employer could encounter criminal charges for their actions.

Fact

Studies show an increased prevalence of migraine among veterans who suffer from PTSD. Veterans who suffer from post-traumatic stress disorder (PTSD) may be able to receive compensation from the Department of Veterans Affairs. Consult your local Veteran Affairs office for more information.

Facing Discrimination

Unfair and illegal though it is, many migraineurs experience discrimination at school and work. Knowing the law helps provide a defense against harassment and discrimination, in the event that it occurs.

One form of discrimination faced by migraineurs is not being allowed enough time for medical appointments. Especially in the early days of diagnosing chronic migraine disease, there is usually a multitude of appointments (scheduled at the doctor's convenience, of course) with physicians, neurologists, and other specialists. Exams such as MRIs or CT scans must be scheduled, and those can take hours depending on how busy the office is on the day of your appointment.

Employers need to allow reasonable amounts of time for an employee to visit the doctor when she is ill. However, do your best to schedule appointments during times when your absence at the office will not disrupt key workflows. Look for after-hours, lunchtime, or early morning appointments. If an appointment must be scheduled in the middle of the workday, try to make sure it does not fall in the middle of an important meeting or conference call. And remember to give your employer plenty of notice, informing him of appointments and estimated time needed away from the office as soon as you have scheduled them.

On-Site Accommodation

There are several ways in which migraineurs can make modifications to their work environments to lessen the impact and discomfort of their disease. However, some employers refuse to make even the most modest of accommodations, citing a disinclination for "special treatment" as a reason for refusal. This behavior constitutes discrimination, and may clearly violate a company's stated antidiscrimination policy, not to mention requirements under the ADA. Read the corporate handbook, know your rights, and insist on fair accommodations per your disability. If your immediate supervisor is not amenable to your needs, do not be afraid to take your concerns to the head of the human resources department or another relevant personnel office.

Essential

Glare-resistant screen coatings, removal of strong perfumes and colognes, and a consistent source of fresh drinking water are small things, but ones that can remove several migraine triggers and contribute to a healthier, trigger-free workday. Another beneficial accommodation would include a quiet room for sleeping in the event of a migraine attack at work.

Chapter 14 has more information on dealing with migraine effectively in the workplace.

Reasonable Time Off

Another way in which migraine sufferers might be discriminated against is in the amount of time they are allowed to take off from work. Some offices have a set number of sick days given to salaried employees; when those days are all gone, so also is the employee's ability to take time out during a migraine attack without having to use vacation hours.

The employer's point of view must be considered. If someone is hired to do a job, and is getting paid to perform the functions of that job, that person is reasonably expected to be in the office doing that job. However, everyone falls ill from time to time, and employers should be willing to make reasonable exceptions for times when an employee is simply unable to function.

If choosing another line of work (one with more flexible hours, for example) is not an option, consider talking to your employer about ways to make up the time. Can you work evenings on the days when your migraine is under control? Can you put in extra hours on the weekend? Coming up with a plan for finishing projects on time, despite the possibility of needing to take a day off when a migraine is at its worst, can go a long way toward building goodwill with employers.

If you work for a public agency, a private or public elementary or secondary school, or a company with more than fifty employees for a period of at least a year, you may also have coverage under the Family and Medical Leave Act (FMLA). The act enables you to take unpaid time off if you experience health problems and your employer does not provide disability or sick-day benefits. It also provides for up to twelve weeks of unpaid leave within a twelve-month period for medical and family caretaking reasons.

Medical Records and Your Rights

Knowing the details of your migraine treatment can be very important to successfully managing the disease. Lab results, medication history, and even doctor's notes are all relevant information, and patients have a right to this knowledge. Attempting to obtain it in a safe and secure manner can raise potential questions and difficulties, however. Do patients really have a right to their complete medical records? What if the doctor refuses to share information with other doctors?

Medical records contain an account of all treatment received from any sort of health professional. Lab results, prescribed medications, surgical history and any other evidence of procedures are included. Complete medical records include your medical history and answers to any questions you may have been asked in the doctor's office, including your pregnancy status and whether or not you smoke, drink, or engage in risky behaviors.

 Fact

If you turn to your doctor for help ascertaining your disabled status, that information becomes part of your medical record as well. In other words, if your diagnosis constitutes that of disability, you can expect that information to live in your record.

National standards were created for the safety, sharing, and protection of medical record information via the HIPAA Privacy Rule of 1996. HIPAA stands for Health Insurance Portability and Accountability Act. Title I provides health insurance coverage when employees lose or change jobs. Title II established standards for electronic records transfer, but also set up rules for PHI (Protected Health Information). Under the law, protected health information consists of any information about a patient that relates to health status or finances. Patients or other covered entities can request updates to incorrect medical data, and confidentiality of medical data must be maintained during transfers.

Getting Access

When it comes to accessing medical records, remember that you are not the only one entitled to your records. A host of others are entitled to see your medical history, including potential employers, Medicare and other government departments, insurance companies, and the Medical Information Bureau. However, remember that under the ADA, employers are not allowed to discriminate on the basis of disability. They cannot, for example, ask potential job applicants for specific information in their medical histories or prescreen employees by requiring physical examinations.

Privacy

Thanks to HIPAA (the Health Insurance Portability and Accountability Act), patient privacy laws became more standardized across the country. Patients have a right to access their medical records, and this access extends to individual health care providers and insurance companies. Oral requests are easy to ignore and impossible to track, so always make a formal request in writing.

 Question

Can marketers gain access to your medical information?
Sometimes, yes. If a person chooses to participate in certain types of public health screenings, for example, that information might be shared or sold. If privacy is a concern, read all printed warnings, waivers, and other documentation before signing on the dotted line.

In addition to the protections provided by the government, be proactive about protecting your privacy. Read waivers carefully and, if necessary, handwrite exceptions onto the form before signing it.

If certain documents in your medical history might initiate conflict at work, for example, ask your doctor to sign a special waiver that removes your consent for sharing that document. Work with your physician and hospital legal department for specific questions and concerns.

Paying for Your Care

Chronic disease is often accompanied by financial hardship. Medical bills accumulate and, if not paid, can be enhanced by interest and possibly legal fees. While shopping around for medical care can be time-consuming and not always in the best interest of the patient, the reality is that you may be able to reduce or eliminate fees altogether with a little bit of research.

You should also be aware that there are both private and public assistance plans available for patients who don't have the financial resources to pay for their own health care and ongoing treatment. These include patient assistance programs that allow low- to no-cost access to prescription medications, and government-sponsored programs.

Flexible Spending Accounts

Most insurance companies will cover the diagnosis and treatment of migraine disease. The exceptions include non-FDA-approved medications and nonformulary medications; some of those expenses may need to be paid out of pocket. To help mitigate these costs, and the cost of any health insurance co-pays, consider opening a Health Care FSA, or Flexible Spending Account. This plan allows working individuals to place pretax dollars into a special account to be used for unreimbursed or uncovered components of medical cost.

FSA accounts can only be opened during specific times of year under most employers' health care plans and must be used completely within a calendar year or the remaining money is forfeited. Talk with the human resources department at your place of work for details.

Work with Your Doctor

What many doctors do not tell patients up front is that fees are often negotiable. If a patient is truly unable to pay for an uncovered procedure, for example, many doctors will reduce their fees. In addition, most doctor's offices and hospitals will provide discounts for cash payments of up to 30 percent, since that is the amount they would forfeit if the account had to be handed to a collection agency. Do not be afraid or embarrassed to ask about fee reductions.

After an expensive procedure, ask to look at an itemized bill. Mistakes in medical billing are common enough that it is worth your time to double-check the amount you are being asked to pay. Follow these basic guidelines when it comes to understanding your bill:

- Make sure the bill is presented to you in writing.
- Only pay for the charges that make sense in plain English and can be explained by the doctor's office.
- Ask questions before paying for any items you don't understand or recognize.
- Only pay for services that you actually received.

Patient Assistance Programs

Most doctors and hospitals provide some amount of charity care, or health care specifically for patients who do not have the means to pay for it. Generally speaking, charity care—which is sometimes called indigent care—is granted depending on the patient's income. Each state and/or institution will have its own formula for calculating eligibility, but broadly speaking, patient income and assets must not exceed a certain percentage of the state's poverty level.

Essential

Patients receiving charity care will not have to pay more than around 25 to 30 percent of their total gross income for medical care. Some states have a fund for charity care, so don't hesitate to ask if your income meets the criteria.

Many pharmaceutical manufacturers also run patient assistance programs that provide low- to no-cost access to prescription drugs. Each company has their own individual application and qualification process. However, the Partnership for Prescription Assistance, an alliance of U.S. drug manufacturers and health care organizations, offers a directory of prescription assistance programs and centralized access to their application procedures at *www.pparx.org*. You can also call their toll-free number for assistance at 1-888-4PPA-NOW.

Dealing with Insurance Issues

While most group health insurance plans cover the diagnoses and treatments relating to migraines, not all insurance is created equal. Also, some insurance plans may not cover preferred doctors or specialists. Research all available options before making an insurance decision.

If you carry your health insurance plan yourself and don't have the support of your company's human resource department to help you determine coverage and fight claim denials, you face additional challenges and obstacles. Become familiar with the health insurance claims and appeals system so you can use the process to your best advantage.

Choosing a Plan

When choosing insurance plans, the first step is to make an accurate estimate of your anticipated medical costs. Look at the Explanation of Benefits from your current policy to see what types of services were covered and at what average costs. Next, obtain your medical records and assign a price to every expenditure; include everything from hospital stays and X-rays to lab tests and prescription medications. Use an average from the past year, or from the past several years if you had unusual medical circumstances arise during one or more years.

The following is a very general guide to costs typically encountered by migraineurs:

- Doctor's visit: Co-pay range $10–$30
- Prescription medication: Co-pay range $10–$20 (generic), $20–$50 (name brand)
- Triptan medications: $20–$70 per dose (out-of-pocket)
- Laboratory tests: $80–$100
- Brief hospitalization: $100–$200 (co-pay), $5,000 (out-of-pocket)
- X-ray or MRI: $300

When considering which insurance plan to choose, there will usually be several options at varying levels of coverage provided by an employer (or more, if insurance is being purchased outside of employment). One of the most important considerations is whether the plans you are considering include the doctors and specialists with whom you want to work. Also, read the general plan description to ensure that all services you anticipate needing are covered.

Essential

Always compare apples to apples when looking at different policies. Compare covered medications and co-pays, as well as premiums, deductibles, and lifetime maximums. Based on your anticipated migraine treatment plan, calculate which plan makes the most economic sense.

Does migraine count as a preexisting medical condition? Generally speaking, the answer is probably yes. Migraine disease is a recognized neurological ailment. Once a diagnosis has been made and becomes part of your medical record, insurance companies have access to that information. If you were covered by one insurance company during migraine treatment, there may be a period of time during which time a new insurance plan will not cover some migraine-related treatment or testing as a "preexisting condition." However, if you have had continuous health insurance coverage for twelve months or more prior to moving to a new insurance plan, the

Health Insurance Portability and Accountability Act (HIPAA) may protect you from a lapse in coverage. Find out if a "preexisting" stipulation will impact your migraine care with a new health insurance plan by speaking with the new insurer before you switch plans. Get any promises or assurances about coverage in writing.

Fighting for Coverage

Suppose you require a procedure from your doctor and, rather than risk a large bill, you choose to presubmit the claim to your insurance company. When the claim is presented, you receive a "denial of coverage" letter and bill for the full cost. Rather than resorting to panic, form a plan to fight back.

First, never assume that the bill you have received is either correct or final; call the insurance company and ask them to explain the bill. If that proves fruitless, ask to speak to a manager and explain why the procedure should be covered under the existing policy. The rule of thumb is that medically necessary procedures should be covered, so make the best argument you can toward that end. Obtain statements from your doctors indicating that the procedure was, in fact, necessary. Any documentation the doctor's office can provide to the insurance company will further your cause.

Speak to the insurance handler with the doctor's office and ask their advice. They may have suggestions for medical billing codes or other insights into how to have the procedure covered. Prepare yourself with evidence showing how other insurance plans cover the same procedure.

If you feel that the insurance representative you reached just doesn't understand the coverage issue at hand, it may help your case and your sanity to end the call. Cool off and regroup, then phone again later and try your luck with someone else. Insurance companies are typically large organizations with a full staff of customer service representatives on hand, and speaking to someone new gives you the opportunity to explain your case again. Remember that no matter what your level of frustration might be at the time, being courteous will only help your case, as customer service representatives almost always respond better to a polite customer than an irritable one.

Insurance companies have an appeals process for denied claims. If coverage is denied, always inquire about the appeals process and start it immediately. Gather any additional information or data from your doctor that you feel might help your case and check back regularly with your insurance company to ensure that the appeal is being processed in a timely manner.

L. Essential

Always document the full names of insurance representatives that you speak with on the phone, in addition to the time and date of the call and the details of what you spoke about. Ask the representative to send you written confirmation of coverage promises and clarifications she makes over the telephone.

Medicare and Migraines

Medicare, the health insurance provided to people age sixty-five and older in the United States, has been administered by law since 1965. All sixty-five-and-over permanent residents (or citizens) of the United States who worked for at least ten years in a Medicare-covered place of work are eligible. In addition, some people younger than sixty-five may be eligible if they are disabled and receive Social Security benefits.

The Basics

Medicare consists of four basic parts:

- Part A: Hospital insurance—states that any hospitalization and nursing home stays longer than three days are covered
- Part B: Medical insurance—states coverage for physician and nursing services, lab tests, flu vaccines, and a host of other procedures

- Part C: Medicare Advantage coverage—states that Medicare recipients can receive their coverage through private health insurance plans
- Part D: Prescription drug coverage—requires enrollment in a Prescription Drug Plan (PDP) or Medicare Advantage with prescription drug coverage

One of the more important things to realize about Medicare is that it does not cover all costs. Medicare patients are still responsible for co-pays, premiums, and deductibles. In order to relieve some of the burden of these out-of-pocket fees, many people choose to also purchase a supplemental coverage plan called Medigap. What Medicare does, however, is allow retired adults with medical conditions such as migraines to continue to receive care and treatment in a similar fashion to their employer-provided health insurance during their working years.

 Fact

Medicare and Medicaid are not the same thing. Medicare is the health insurance provided to individuals aged sixty-five and over. Medicaid is health insurance for low-income individuals and families. Medicaid has been in existence since 1965 and is funded by both states and the federal government.

As with any other large, government-run program, Medicare is a system that can be confusing and full of bureaucracy. With the recent availability of private health plans and prescription drug coverage for Medicare recipients, the number of choices, and therefore the potential for confusion, is higher than ever. However, with an investment of time, or the help of a trained Medicare advocate, migraineurs can find coverage that allows them to receive high-quality medical care and appropriate prescription drugs.

Part D Drug Coverage

When choosing a Prescription Drug Plan, remember that not all plans cover the same medications. To choose a PDP that will cover your migraine medications, start by making a list of the medications you currently take. Consider dosages and how many pills you take per month. Next, look at the Standard Benefit for the different PDPs you are considering to get a sense for how deductibles will work when compared to the amount you expect to spend on migraine and other medications each year.

There are a vast number of plans available, and they will all be competing for your business. The best way to make an educated decision is to consult an expert; the AARP (American Association of Retired Persons) and Medicare both offer online tools to compare drug plans and search for particular prescription drugs. Remember that there is an annual enrollment period for Medicare Part D Drug Coverage, so research and make choices well in advance of the deadline.

CHAPTER 19

Beyond Migraine: Comorbidities

A NUMBER OF conditions and diseases are found in conjunction with migraines, emphasizing the complex interactions between migraines and other systems of the body. Comorbidity refers to an association of two disorders in the same person, one that is more frequent than could be explained by pure coincidence. Some diseases often found to be comorbid, or coexisting, with migraines include stroke, depression, epilepsy, asthma, and Raynaud's disease. Because some migraine drugs may either help or aggravate comorbid conditions, and vice versa, your doctor must create a treatment plan that will address your whole health picture.

Comorbidities: An Overview

Why certain health conditions appear more frequently alongside migraine disease is not completely understood. But the comorbidity between migraines and other conditions such as stroke and epilepsy may be based on one of four links:

- Coincidental
- Causative, where one disorder causes the other
- Etiologically based, with a genetic or environmental link between the two disorders
- Etiologically based, where a particular physical state results in both disorders

Treating Two Conditions

The best treatment for migraine and a comorbid condition is often to find a drug that has had proven success in the treatment of both conditions. Care must be taken to ensure that a drug that treats one condition, like migraine, is not contraindicated for another condition. For example, beta-blockers (which are commonly used to treat migraine) should not be used on patients with asthma even though they are comorbid conditions.

In addition, doctors must be careful that drugs being taken for comorbid conditions do not cause or trigger migraines and that there are no harmful drug interactions between a migraine medication and the other drugs that a patient may be taking. The goal, then, is finding a drug that will safely treat both the migraine and the comorbid disease. Since many innovations in migraine treatment come from off-label use of preexisting drugs, there are a number of drugs initially intended for other conditions that have proven successful in treating migraines. These drugs are a natural starting point if a patient is found to have a comorbidity with a relevant condition.

Stroke and Cardiovascular Disease

A 2006 study published in the *Journal of the American Medical Association* found that active migraines with aura in women were associated with an increased risk of cardiovascular disease, including myocardial infarction, stroke, angina, and death. Interestingly, active migraines without aura in women were not found to be correlated with any increased risk of cardiovascular disease. It is theorized that the same vascular problems that cause migraines could also extend to the coronary arteries, increasing the risk of heart attacks and other events.

It can be hard to determine the exact relationship between migraine and stroke because the timing of a stroke with respect to the onset of a migraine is rarely recorded with any degree of accuracy. There does seem to be an increased risk of ischemic stroke for women diagnosed with migraines who are under forty-five years old, as reported by the *British Journal of Medicine* in 1993. A 1989 study in the journal *Acta Neurologica Scandinavica* also found that between 1 and 17 percent of strokes in patients less than fifty years old had an association with migraines.

Cholesterol Connection

A 2005 study in *Neurology* found an association between patients with migraine and patients with symptoms of heart disease. Patients who had migraine with aura were found to be 43 percent more likely to have high cholesterol than the general population, and they were 76 percent more likely to have high blood pressure. Such patients had a higher risk from the effects of heart disease with age, and reported a fourfold increase in the incidence of stroke or heart disease before they reached the age of forty-five.

It's important to note that migraineurs are also more likely to smoke, which is a major risk factor for heart disease and stroke. The Norweigan Head-HUNT study found that prevalance rates for headache were higher among smokers compared with those who have never smoked. And a study published in 2008 in the journal *Headache* found that individuals who suffered from frequent headaches during mid-adolescence were twice as likely to smoke in adulthood than those without headache.

Platelet Dysfunction

Another study, from the *Journal of Neurology, Neurosurgery, and Psychiatry* in 2004, suggests that a link could exist between stroke and migraines on a more fundamental level. A platelet dysfunction, in which proinflammatory platelets adhere to leukocytes, has been observed in stroke patients. A similar process has been observed in migraine patients. It is thought that this dysfunction takes place during the interval in between migraine attacks, when the patient is headache free. It is possible, therefore, that there is a connection between migraines and strokes on a level as fundamental as the interactions between single cells. Future study is needed to determine if there are other biochemical links between the two conditions.

Complex Relationships

The overall occurrence of a stroke during or immediately follow-ing a migraine attack is fortunately a rare event. A 2003 study in the journal *Archives of Neurology* describes two cases in which patients suffered from "migrainous infarction." In these cases, pathogenesis appeared in some way as a direct result of the migraine and took place during the course of a normal migraine with aura. The exact nature of the relationship between stroke and migraine in this cir-cumstance is unknown.

 Fact

A study in the New England Journal of Medicine mentions that 26 percent of patients with a particular type of angina, related to coronary artery spasm, also had migraines, as compared to 6 percent of patients with a more typical presentation of coronary artery disease (and 10 percent of the general population).

A complex relationship seems to exist between migraine and stroke. In cases where a stroke occurs in a migraineur that is unrelated to a recent or current migraine, it is likely that the co-occurrence is either coincidental or is due to shared risk factors. Another category of interrelationship is when a structural cerebral defect is found that can produce the clinical signs of a migraine, or when a stroke happens to include a migraine-like headache that is unrelated to any typical migraine triggers or patterns. It is only when a stroke occurs during or immediately following a migraine that the migraine can be considered to have caused the stroke, and only after all other possible causes of the stroke have been ruled out.

Treatments

Beta-blockers or calcium channel blockers can successfully treat patients who have hypertension or angina along with migraines. Sumatriptan (Imitrex) and other "triptan" drugs should not be taken by patients who have previously had a myocardial infarction, heart disease, or angina, or who have hypertension that is not controlled. Beta-blockers should not be used in migraine patients who also have hypotension (low blood pressure), diabetes, or asthma.

Depression

Depression is another common condition linked to migraines. A 2000 study in the journal *Neurology* showed that people with migraines or other serious headache conditions are three times more likely to experience a major depression than the general population. Similarly, a 1994 study in the journal *Headache* found that patients with a history of major depression are 3.1 times more likely to experience the initiation of migraines than those without a history of depression.

 Fact

A major Canadian health survey published in 2007 found that migraineurs experienced comorbid depression, bipolar disorder, panic disorder, and social phobia twice as often as those without migraine, and migraineurs with psychiatric comorbidities had poorer health outcomes. However, migraine was not associated with an increased incidence of substance or alcohol abuse.

These results, though powerful, do not necessarily suggest a cause-and-effect relationship between depression and migraine, or migraine and depression. The correlation between migraine and mood disorders such as depression could be rooted in the stress that comes from dealing with either condition. More likely, however, some underlying biological predisposition sets the stage for both conditions, creating the appearance of an association between the two.

Crossover Medications

Some drugs are available that can treat both conditions. If sleep is also disrupted due to the depression and migraines, the drug of choice may be an antidepressant such as amitriptyline (Elavil). This drug serves to help regulate the serotonergic pathways and treats both depression and migraine separately. At the same time, this drug may help with sleep disruptions, as it can be very sedating. However, amitriptyline can have other adverse side effects, and other similar drugs with less bothersome side effects, such as nortriptyline (Pamelor) are prescribed instead. Beta-blockers should not be used to treat migraines in patients who suffer from depression.

Selective serotonin reuptake inhibitors (SSRIs) have also been used to treat patients who suffer from both migraine and depression, but such drugs have shown only limited efficacy in clinical trials. Such drugs may be prescribed by physicians who believe that stress and anxiety can trigger migraines. Monoamine oxidase inhibitors (MAOIs) are also sometimes used for patients who suffer from depression as well as migraine.

Epilepsy

Like stroke and depression, migraine and epilepsy have a well-documented association. Individuals with migraine or epilepsy are more than twice as likely to have the other condition. While the prevalence of epilepsy in the general population is only 0.5 to 1 percent, in migraineurs it is about 5.9 percent. Similarly, the Epilepsy Family Study of Columbia University found that 24 percent of people with epilepsy have been found to have migraines, compared with only 12 percent of the general population.

It has been found that the age of first seizure is unrelated to the risk of developing migraines, suggesting that migraines are not solely responsible for epilepsy and also not the sole result. It is possible that there are subtle alterations in brain chemistry, such as lower levels of magnesium, changes in neurotransmitter levels, or other possible complex biological factors that could simultaneously increase the risk of both migraine and epilepsy.

Common Factors

Despite being distinct conditions, epilepsy and migraine share a surprising number of commonalities. They are both episodic, chronic, neurological disorders. A 2005 study in the journal *Advanced Studies in Medicine* reports that a migraine with visual aura may be difficult to distinguish from an epileptic seizure with visual hallucinations, and migraines can cause an altered state of partial consciousness that is similar to a complex partial epileptic seizure. Visual symptoms show the most similarities between the two conditions. They occur in 15 to 20 percent of patients with a migraine, but occur in only 5 to 8 percent of epileptic seizures.

Altered consciousness is also a common symptom between the two conditions; it is found only in rare subtypes of migraines but takes place in about 40 percent of seizures. Even headache, which might seem to indicate a migraine by definition, is not a definitive diagnostic tool. The 2005 study reports that up to 20 percent of migraine auras may occur in isolation from a headache, while as many as 19 percent of patients with epilepsy report a headache during the course of, or following, a seizure.

The study suggests that electroencephalography (EEG) may be one of the few ways to quantitatively distinguish between an epileptic seizure and a migraine when they share these common manifestations.

In a migraine, the EEG usually appears normal, though some focal slowing may be present. During a seizure, however, the EEG usually shows a typical seizure pattern, although simple partial seizures may be mild enough not to have a diagnostic seizure pattern easily visible on the EEG. Therefore, while EEG is a useful tool to distinguish between some migraines and seizures, it is not completely reliable.

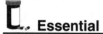

Essential

Since migraine and epilepsy are comorbid and often occur together, techniques like EEG may be necessary to supplement a clinical diagnosis. EEG is a common tool used to diagnose epilepsy but is rarely used on migraineurs.

Treatments for Epilepsy and Migraine

In addition to having some similar characteristics, migraine and epilepsy are also frequently found together in the same patient. For example, one migraine variation, familial hemiplegic migraine, is often associated with epilepsy, although the manifestation of each is different enough to allow separate diagnoses. As in other migraine comorbidities, it is often advantageous to the patient to find a drug that can treat both migraine and epilepsy simultaneously.

Fact

Other neurological problems are sometimes comorbid with migraines, and can have similar treatments to epilepsy. For example, the treatments described for epilepsy are often also effective for patients who have bipolar or manic depressive illness as well as a prophylaxis for migraines.

Some drugs primarily intended to treat epilepsy have shown to be very effective in treating migraines as well. Divalproex sodium (Depakote) and topiramate (Topamax) are indicated by the FDA as effective in treatment for both epilepsy and migraines. Chapter 8 has more information on antiepileptic drugs, or AEDs, used to treat migraine.

Asthma

There have been reported links between migraine and asthma. Studies such as a recent one published in the *British Journal of General Practice* have demonstrated that patients with migraine disease tend to display symptoms of asthma, including nonseasonal wheezing and breathing difficulty. Those formally diagnosed with chronic migraines are more likely to experience adult onset of asthma.

 Alert

The correlation between asthma and migraine appears to be inherited. Children having parents with migraine disease are as much as five times more likely to be diagnosed with asthma. Parents with migraines should be extra cautious about having their children examined for asthma at the first sign of wheezing or breathing difficulty.

While the exact cause of the connection between migraine and asthma is not known, the predominant theory is that it is muscular in nature. There is an airway smooth muscle (ASM) that, when narrowed, seems to lead to asthma flare-ups. Similarly, blood vessel walls contain smooth muscle, and there is a theory that the inflammation of that muscle leads to vasoconstriction, or narrowing of the blood vessels. Whether simultaneous muscle contraction occurs or one type of contraction influences the other is not clear. Further research is needed to explore the relationship and possible commonalities between migraine and asthma.

 Fact

Beta-blockers should not be used to treat migraines in patients who suffer from asthma. An alternative migraine treatment for asthma patients is calcium antagonists such as verapamil and flunarizine.

As with migraine, asthma is treated through both abortive and preventative medication. Quick-relief drugs are those that help restore breathing in the midst of an asthma attack; these medications include beta-2 agonists that act as bronchodilators. Preventative drugs are taken daily and help prevent the incidence of asthma attack; inhaled corticosteroids and long-acting beta-2 agonists are common medications in this class.

Raynaud's Disease

Raynaud's disease causes the extremities (toes, fingers, and the tips of the nose and ears) to feel cold or numb. It tends to flare up in either cold weather or under stressful conditions. There is a known correlation between patients with migraine and Raynaud's disease. Migraine sufferers have a higher tendency to be diagnosed with Raynaud's disease; the reverse statement is also true.

Pathology

When a person has Raynaud's disease, the arteries near the skin tend to constrict. As a result, blood flow to the extremities is lessened, hence the feeling of coldness and numbness. As blood supply to those extremities is compromised, the skin may turn white or pale colored. If oxygen flow lessens considerably, those same areas may turn blue.

 Question

Why are Raynaud's disease patients more likely to also have migraine disease?
The precise connection between Raynaud's disease and migraine is not known. Migraine sufferers often report heightened sensitivity to cold and tingling in their fingers. Also, both diseases involve reactivity of the blood vessels in response to some trigger, suggesting that common factors are at play.

Note that Raynaud's disease flare-ups are episodic. In times of cold weather, flare-ups may occur. Once the skin is warmed, blood flow to those regions returns and skin color should become more normal.

Migraine Similarities

In both migraine and Raynaud's disease, the vascular system is often more reactive than in normal patients, and vasomotor instability is common. Raynaud's flare-ups are fairly predictable—that is, they occur with a change in temperature. Migraine attacks can be predictable once triggers are identified, but they can also strike seemingly at random. To that end, Raynaud's disease may be easier for patients to manage.

Treatment for Raynaud's and Migraine

For patients who suffer from migraines and Raynaud's disease, calcium channel blocking drugs such as verapamil (Calan, Isoptin) are commonly given. These drugs are preventative, and must be taken for many weeks or even months before the full benefit can be seen. Beta-adrenergic antagonist drugs, or beta-blockers such as propranolol, are widely used to help prevent migraines, but should not be used for patients who have Raynaud's disease because they can make circulation problems worse.

Other Conditions

There are several other conditions that have an association with migraines. It is thought that because of the prevalence of both diseases occurring in individual patients, this association is more than coincidence, making them other potential comorbidities.

A short list of these potential associations includes:

- Endometriosis
- Essential tremor

- Generalized anxiety disorder
- Insomnia and sleep disorders
- Irritable bowel syndrome
- Mitral valve prolapse
- Multiple sclerosis
- Panic disorder
- Patent foramen ovale
- Simple and social phobia
- Systemic lupus erythematosus

Diagnosis and Treatment

Headache is often one of the initial symptoms of multiple sclerosis. A 2004 study published in the journal *Cephalgia* found that over half of MS patients studied experienced headache, and 25 percent of the MS study population had diagnosed migraine. The same MRI abnormalities found in multiple sclerosis can also be found in migraine, making an accurate diagnosis sometimes difficult. One University of Colorado study of 281 patients referred for further workup because of suspected MS found that 37 percent of these patients actually had migraine instead.

Migraine is also associated with sleep disorders such as insomnia. A broader category of such issues is parasomnias, which refers to undesired physical phenomena that occur during sleep. Several studies have found higher levels of parasomnias in children with migraine than in children without the condition. Parasomnias such as night terrors (known clinically as *pavor nocturnus*) are more prevalent in migraineurs than in the general population. A French study of children with migraine found that 56 percent of patients, as opposed to 16 percent of controls, experience sleepwalking. And a survey of parents found that 41 percent of pediatric migraineurs experienced enuresis (bed-wetting) as opposed to 16 percent of children without migraine.

Though not as common, these conditions may also be treated by drugs that are also effective on migraine. For example, essential tremor can be treated by beta-blockers and topiramate, drugs that are also effective for migraines. And tricyclic antidepressants can be effective in treatment of insomnia as well as migraine. Make sure that the physician who treats your migraines is aware of any preexisting health conditions and the drugs you take for them.

CHAPTER 20

The Future of Migraine Care

IN AN IDEAL world, migraine would not exist. Given that it does, however, the ultimate goal for migraine sufferers and caretakers is to reduce symptoms to the point where migraineurs can lead fulfilling and normal lives. In a sense, the goal of the future of migraine care should be to stop migraines before they begin with the aid of medications that are safe to take for long periods of time and that have no serious side effects. Other new and exciting options for migraine care include innovations in therapeutic procedures, as well as taking advantage of cutting-edge treatment via clinical trials.

Drugs in the Pipeline

One of the most encouraging aspects of current migraine therapy is that there is always room for improvement. New medications are constantly being studied and tested. The cream of the crop will eventually be available for the general public, but in the meantime, here is a preview of some medications that one day may make an appearance at a pharmacy near you.

MK-0974

A new medication, currently called MK-0974, has been wowing researchers. This is a different class of drug from the triptans that many migraine sufferers take, but it has the possibility of working for those who cannot tolerate triptans. The idea behind MK-0974 is that it inhibits the release of calcitonin gene-related peptide (CGRP), which is a protein that is released during inflammation; migraineurs are often seen to have high levels of this protein.

One advantage of this drug is that it would be safer for patients with heart disease because it does not make blood vessels constrict. Early studies show the possibility of MK-0974 success in patients who, for any number of reasons, are unable to achieve relief from triptans. Early reports indicate that as many as 65 percent of people who try MK-0974 report decreased migraine pain. This drug needs further testing before it can be made available to the general public, but watch for news about it in the next few years.

Botox

Botox has been in the news in recent years for its ability to temporarily reduce the appearance of facial wrinkles. However, new research shows that it may also be valuable as a treatment for migraine. Botulinum toxin type A, or Botox (BTX-A), is a toxin that is most commonly injected into muscles to cause a decrease in muscle activity. However, studies show that when injected into the upper portion of the face, Botox has the potential to reduce the incidence of migraine for up to six months.

While the discovery of Botox's applicability to migraine was accidental, researchers seized on this information and began looking for confirmation. As yet, Botox is not an FDA-approved treatment for migraine. For this reason, the treatment is not covered by most insurance policies. See Chapter 8 for more information on botulism A as a migraine preventative.

Trexima

Another new medication that has the potential to relieve migraine pain is called Trexima. This is a combination therapy, one that combines Imitrex with naproxen sodium. Naproxen sodium is a nonsteroidal anti-inflammatory drug; the version available over the counter in the United States is called Aleve. Trexima is currently under FDA review, and has shown positive results in reducing migraine pain.

Alternate Delivery

Many child migraine sufferers, and some adults, have difficult swallowing tablets. In addition, the nausea and vomiting that often accompanies a migraine attack can make keeping down medication a challenge.

Some newer versions of migraine medications are available in nasal spray form, and these have the potential to make abortive drugs more widely accepted and easier to tolerate. One example is Sumatriptan nasal spray, which comes with a simple delivery mechanism that is both effective and child-friendly. Nasal sprays are fast acting and ensure that the maximum dose can be absorbed.

There are also new needle-free injection systems coming down the pipeline, including Intraject. This system features subcutaneous injections that are painless and easy. Lingual spray systems for Sumatriptan are also being developed, as are meltable tablets and sustained-release patches.

Transcranial Magnetic Stimulation (TMS)

One of the most exciting developments in future migraine care, Transcranial Magnetic Stimulation (TMS) is a method of stimulating the brain using electromagnets. The theory behind using TMS with migraine care is that, according to research, the brains of migraine patients tend to have different levels of excitability during migraine attacks, as opposed to when the migraineur is attack free. TMS can both investigate changes in brain activity as well as excite areas of the brain. Currently being used to diagnose diseases such as stroke and multiple sclerosis and to research the impact of neurological conditions like migraine on the brain, TMS has the potential to also be used therapeutically in the future.

History and Mechanism

The idea of using electromagnetic induction to influence brain activity has been around for hundreds of years. Since at least the eighteenth century, scientists have been experimenting with electromagnets and electric currents. That research led to the idea of using electrodes to stimulate muscles; by the mid-nineteenth century, physicians such as Roberts Bartholow began to make headway in using electric currents to excite areas of the human brain. Further research and experiments were conducted over the years, with some of the first distinctly TMS therapies occurring in the 1980s.

When TMS is used as therapy, magnetic pulses are created with an electromagnet attached to the patient's scalp. Pulses are sent in one of two methods: single or repetitive. Single short pulses stimulate the cerebral cortex, thereby altering patterns of brain activity for short periods of time. Repetitive pulses (rTMS) have the tendency to produce longer-acting effects.

TMS is considered a noninvasive procedure. Anesthesia is not used, and the electromagnet is painlessly attached to the scalp. Patients who have received TMS report hearing a slight tapping sound. Muscle contraction is another side effect, as the brain stimulation can affect areas in the scalp, face, and jaw.

While a small number (5 to 10 percent) of patients experienced discomfort at the site where the electromagnet was attached, most reported the experience to be pain free. When used therapeutically, most patients received daily half-hour sessions. These sessions were maintained for anywhere between two to six weeks.

 Question

Is Transcranial Magnetic Stimulation only considered beneficial to migraine sufferers?
No, TMS is being researched for its application to many illnesses. In addition to migraine, early studies have shown the possibility for TMS to be helpful in treating depression, hallucination, Parkinson's disease, and tinnitus.

Potential Risks and Treatment

Because of the nature of the brain stimulation, TMS has the potential to cause seizures. However, this incidence is rare (especially with low-frequency doses), and there have not been serious cases of seizure reported. However, since TMS is not an FDA-approved procedure as of this writing, joining a trial or volunteering for research are the only ways to currently take advantage of TMS treatment.

Preliminary studies conducted at Ohio State University showed that TMS had the ability to significantly (by up to 69 percent) reduce the pain and intensity of an active migraine attack. This study also showed that after receiving TMS, migraine sufferers reported significantly less sensitivity to noise and light, in addition to being relieved of their nausea. Further research is required in order to prove a definitive correlation between migraine relief and TMS, but early studies look promising.

Occipital Nerve Stimulation

For those who do not object to having a device implanted in their brain, Occipital Nerve Stimulation for the Treatment of Intractable Migraine (ONSTIM) may one day be a treatment option. While not commercially available or FDA approved, this futuristic treatment offers a new type of potential relief.

So far, this technique has only been tried in a few clinical trials on a small number of patients. Individuals who participated in the ONSTIM trial had a neurostimulator implanted underneath their skin, near the base of the head. The purpose of the neurostimulator is to send electrical impulses to the occipital nerves; these are delivered through wires that are placed underneath the skin. In the trials, the implant was only approved for people for whom other medications provide insufficient relief from migraine recurrence.

After placement of the device, participants noted decreases in migraine pain of up to 50 percent. When tested on individuals who experienced cluster headaches, similar results were achieved. While this percentage is appealing, note that Occipital Nerve Stimulation is not a noninvasive procedure, and only appeared to be effective for certain patients. Results also indicated that the effects were short-lived, and that headaches returned once the stimulator was turned off. While the preliminary form of this treatment may not be ready for commercial sale, its limited success is sure to initiate future research.

⌶ Essential

Neurostimulation comes in one of two forms. Internal neurostimulation involves surgically implanted neurostimulators, along with batteries and leads. Internal/external neurostimulation involves implanting the stimulator and leads, but batteries are worn outside the body.

Identifying Genetic Connections

Genetic influence on migraine is very strong. Migraines tend to run in families, and estimates suggest that a person with a parent who has migraines has a 40 to 50 percent chance of also developing them. A person with migraines has a 70 to 80 percent chance of having a close family member (parent or sibling) who also has them. The results can also be divided into migraine with and without aura. First-degree relatives of those having migraine with aura have a chance of developing migraine with aura themselves that is four times greater than the general population. Correspondingly, such relatives of those having migraine without aura are 1.9 times more likely to develop migraine without aura.

Genetic studies suggest that multiple genes are involved in triggering migraines. A 2007 study in the journal *Archives of Neurology*, for example, found that three different genes—CACNA1A; ATP1A2; and SCN1A—play a role in one rare type of migraine called familial hemiplegic migraine (FHM). Since there is such variation in how migraines are experienced, as well as symptoms and triggers, it seems likely that many different genes are responsible.

Alert

A study in the journal Cephalalgia found that identical twins had higher chances of both having migraines when compared with fraternal twins. However, the rate for identical twins was not 100 percent, indicating that it is not only genetic factors that influence the development of migraine. The environment must be involved as well.

Combined Factors

It is suspected that a number of genes, working separately or together, combine to result in a lowered threshold to common migraine triggers. Future models of the genetic contribution to migraines will not only help illuminate the complex series of mechanisms through which migraines are triggered, but also help produce new therapies and prophylactic targets for migraine treatment.

Identifying Commonalities

Current research using genetically modified mice is helping researchers to pinpoint the specific mechanisms at play in migraine initiation, as well as target particular genes for intervention by new drug therapies. In the case of familial hemiplegic migraine, it appears that all three genes work together to increase the concentration of extracellular neurotransmitters in the brain. This increased concentration causes hyperexcitation of the neurons, as well as a decrease in the threshold for cortical spreading depression (CSD).

Fact

Familial hemiplegic migraine is a rare form of migraine that causes weakness in one side of the body during the aura phase. It may also be accompanied by ataxia, or gross incoordination of muscle movement. It is called familial because part of the diagnostic criteria is an immediate family history of the condition.

CSD is a known trigger of migraine aura, the precursor to many migraines. While these studies have been done only on one particular subclass of migraine, researchers believe that the results can be generalized to more common forms of migraine as well, since FHM migraines have an aura and headache that are very similar to common migraines. FHM patients and relatives are also at increased risk for normal migraines with aura, suggesting that the two types of migraine likely have some pathways in common.

In addition, the three genes implicated in the FHM study all are transporters of ions, leading researchers to believe that disruptions in ions are prevalent in FHM and normal migraines. As studies like these begin to identify the molecular basis of migraines and the metabolic pathways that are involved, researchers will gain a better understanding of the genetic basis for migraine triggers. Future preventative therapies will be able to target the specific mechanisms that trigger migraines.

Clinical Trials—Are They for You?

One of the best ways to receive cutting-edge treatment, often at no cost, is through a clinical trial. For diseases with rapidly evolving treatments, sometimes the only way to use the latest medication or take advantage of the latest procedure is by joining a trial. Furthermore, you can be part of medical history by contributing to a clinical trial; without trials, most medications would never have enough proof of success to be approved by the FDA and, in the process, be made available to wide audiences.

Clinical trials are, by definition, health research studies that follow established protocols. Qualified individuals can participate as long as they meet the "inclusion criteria." Criteria can include medical history, age, gender and details on their form of the disease being treated. Not all qualified applicants will be accepted into any given clinical trial.

Considerations

Many people wonder how safe it is to participate in a clinical trial. Participants must understand that while the FDA and the study leaders make every effort to ensure a safe and profitable experience, some risks are inherent in the process of trying out untested medications and procedures. Careful reading of the study literature, as well as the documents provided as part of informed consent, should make participants feel comfortable with the level of risk they may be taking.

Fact

There are several different types of clinical trials. They include treatment trials (for testing experimental medications and surgeries), diagnostic trials (to test procedures and diagnostic tools), screening trials (where methods of screening for various diseases are examined) and prevention trials (for learning new ways of preventing disease).

All individuals accepted into a clinical trial will sign a consent form. In providing informed consent, patients state that they have had the opportunity to learn the major elements of the study, and have made knowledgeable decisions about whether or not to participate. Generally speaking, participants can withdraw from clinical trials at any point during the process, although their own treatment results might be affected or compromised.

What to Expect

When deciding whether or not to take part in a clinical trial, individuals should consider several factors:

- The nature and purpose of the study
- Why the study is being conducted, and results of similar studies

- The doctors and other health professionals running the study and providing patient care
- The length and requirements of the trial
- Any costs involved with participating, as well as other reimbursable expenses
- Follow-up care after completion of the study

All clinical trials are different in terms of the details of the study protocols. Most begin with a physical and/or psychiatric examination. Participants receive instructions, including how often they need to present themselves at the medical facility or hospital. There are usually strict rules for participants to follow, and individuals can expect to be ejected from the study if they prove incapable of adhering to those guidelines. Generally, most clinical trials allow participants to continue working with their own personal physicians.

Fact

Before a drug can enter clinical trials, it must undergo extensive preclinical testing, which includes animal and in vitro (or lab) study. That may be followed by phase 0 trials, in which 10 to 15 human subjects are given subtherapeutic doses of a drug to gather very basic data on its pharmaceutical action.

Clinical trials for drug testing consist of several phases:

- **Phase I:** a relatively small sampling of participants test an experimental medication, treatment, or procedure, most often in an attempt to identify doses of the drug that are potentially effective yet free of potentially toxic side effects.
- **Phase II:** after the Phase I dose is determined, the trial group is expanded to a larger group of people to test whether the drug shows actual effectiveness in treating the condition in question.

- **Phase III:** the trial group is expanded again, but this time the trial group is divided into one or more groups in which one group will receive the trial drug, and another group will receive a comparison drug or often a placebo, a pill or procedure made to look like the drug or procedure being tested. The assignment to these different groups is random so participants in one of these phase III trials may be as likely to receive the trial drug as a placebo. This procedure is absolutely necessary to confirm the effectiveness of a new treatment; many studies have shown that patients with a variety of conditions, especially migraine, can often respond quite effectively to placebo.
- **Phase IV:** studies are performed after a drug or treatment has made it to market in order to assess the efficacy of a treatment in the larger population of patients and to determine the occurrence of any side effects associated with long-term use.

Study participants may or may not be paid for their participation in a clinical trial. The trials that pay are typically the ones with less of a chance of medical benefit to the subject, since there is an underlying assumption that those trials may have a harder time attracting qualified applicants. Also, payment usually correlates to the length of the study, requirements upon the participant, and expected level of discomfort as a result of study medications or procedures.

Risks and Benefits

One of the primary benefits of participating in a clinical trial is getting access to new treatments before they are available to the general population. Trial participants typically can work with medical experts in their field, and they have the side benefit of knowing that they are playing an important role in medical history.

Clinical trials are, however, not without their risks. Some medications being studied could have unpleasant side effects, and the study could be more draining than the participant anticipated. In addition, there is always the possibility that the therapy being tested by the trial will not help.

Essential

Even trials that do not pay participants almost always provide the required tests, medications, and other examinations or treatments at no cost to participants. They often also reimburse participants for travel expenses to and from the hospital or clinic.

Not everyone who takes part in a clinical trial will have the opportunity to test new medications or therapies. When you take part in a phase III randomized and blinded controlled trial, there is the possibility that you will be assigned to the control group, or the group of study subjects that do not receive the treatment being tested and instead receive a placebo. If the study is blinded, you will not know which group you are in. Keep in mind that even if you do end up in the control group, you are still playing a vital role in medical research.

Locating Trials

There are several ways to locate clinical trials. Working directly with special interest groups responsible for various trials is the best way to find a trial in a specific field. The U.S. National Institutes of Health has a database of clinical trials, sorted by topic. The listings include almost 50,000 trials in over a hundred different countries. The migraine list can be found at: *www.clinicaltrials .gov/search/term=Migraine*

Another clinical trial listing service can be found at Center Watch: *www.centerwatch.com/patient/studies/cat100.html* which also has a listing for pediatric migraine clinical studies: *www.centerwatch.com/ patient/studies/cat440.html*

Advances in Migraine Diagnosis

It is undeniable that there have been vast advances in migraine diagnosis over the years. Much of the recent rise in the numbers of those afflicted with migraine disease is attributable to better diagnostics.

A century ago, migraine sufferers were largely a silent population. Their seemingly erratic behavior led others to consider them eccentric or insane, and in some cases they were thought to be alcoholics or drug addicts. Now that migraine disease is easier to diagnose, those suffering from the disease have many more options available for treatment.

Symptom Awareness

Perhaps the single most important factor in modern migraine diagnosis is the fact that medical professionals are trained in recognizing the symptoms. "A really bad headache" is one clue, but now it is well established that noise and light sensitivity, nausea and vomiting, visual disturbances and dizziness are all common symptoms of a migraine. The ease with which doctors can recognize these symptoms allows for faster and more accurate diagnoses.

In recent years, migraines were easily confused with other types of headaches. Sinus headache, tension headache, cluster headache, and migraine all share similar components, so their confusion is understandable. However, as medical professionals have learned more about migraine-specific symptoms, correct diagnoses allow for significantly better treatment. Sinus headaches will not respond to triptan medication; conversely, a migraine is generally not relieved with saline spray and steam. Learning to distinguish and isolate headache characteristics has been a tremendous boon for migraineurs and their ability to obtain effective treatment.

Differential Diagnosis

While migraine is very difficult to confirm using modern diagnostic and imaging equipment, these tests are invaluable in ensuring that a migraine is not in fact a more life-threatening condition.

Electroencephalogram (EEG) can show brain malfunction, CT and magnetic resonance imaging (MRI) scans can identify brain tumors and many other abnormalities. When someone experiences "the worst headache of her life," diagnostic neuroimaging can be a life-saving procedure.

Additional Resources

General Migraine Information

National Headache Foundation, 1-888-NHF-5552
✑ *www.headaches.org*

American Headache Society Committee for Headache Education (includes physician finder)
✑ *www.achenet.org*

Everything Migraines
✑ *www.everythingmigraines.com*

Help for Headaches with Teri Robert
✑ *www.helpforheadaches.com*

The International Headache Society
✑ *www.i-h-s.org*

National Institute of Neurological Disorders and Stroke (NINDS), the National Institutes of Health
✑ *www.ninds.nih.gov*

Finding Your Health Care Team

American Academy of Neurology (AAN), 800-879-1960
✑ *www.aan.com*

Association for Applied Psychophysiology and Biofeedback (AAPB)
✍ *www.aapb.org*

National Headache Foundation (NHF), free listing of NHF physician members, 1-888-643-5552
MAGNUM Regional Migraine and Headache Clinics
✍ *www.migraines.org/help/helpclin.htm*

Advocacy Organizations

National Headache Foundation, 1-888-NHF-5552
✍ *www.headaches.org*

MAGNUM (Migraine Awareness Group: A National Understanding for Migraineurs), The National Migraine Association
✍ *www.migraines.org*

Patient Assistance Programs

The Pharmaceutical Research and Manufacturers of American (PhRMA), 1-888-4PPA-NOW
✍ *www.helpingpatients.org*

Support Groups

National Headache Foundation support group finder
✍ *www.headaches.org/NHF_Programs/Support_Groups*

Migraines Yahoo Group
✍ *health.groups.yahoo.com/group/migraine*

Daily Strength Migraine Support
✍ *www.dailystrength.org/support-groups/Brain_Nervous_
System/Migraine_Headaches*

Sample Headache Diary

Date _____

Time _____

Prodromal Symptoms

- Aura
- Tingling or numbness
- Difficulty concentrating
- Mood changes
- Photophobia (sensitivity to light)
- Other _____

Head Pain

- Intensity_____
- Location _____
- Description (e.g., stabbing, throbbing)
  _____
  _____
  _____
  _____
  _____

Other Symptoms

- Nausea
- Vomiting
- Sensitivity to light
- Sensitivity to sound
- Sensitivity to odor

Triggers

- Food and beverages
- Drugs
- Weather
- Physical activity
- Lighting
- Sounds
- Odors
- Travel
- Date of last menstrual cycle
- Other _____

Medication

- Name and dosage ____
  _____
- When taken _____
- Effectiveness _____

Other Comfort Measures

- Rest/Sleep
- Compresses
- Progressive relaxation
- Biofeedback
- Other _____

Outcome

- Duration of migraine
  _____
  _____
  _____
- Efficacy of treatment
  _____
  _____
  _____
- Other _____
  _____
  _____
  _____

Postdromal Symptoms

- Mental confusion
- Fatigue
- Weakness
- Lingering head pain
- Mood change
- Other _____
  _____
  _____
  _____

Impact on Quality of Life

- Work missed?
- Work interference?
- Social or family
  obligations missed?
- Other _____
  _____
  _____
  _____

Emergency Patient Forms

Emergency Migraine Treatment Form

I am currently experiencing a severe migraine headache attack. This form contains information about my migraine history, my prescribed treatments, and my health insurance. I am not a substance abuser or "drug seeker." I have attached a document from my physician that verifies my diagnosis and current treatment. Thank you for your assistance.

Patient Information

Name _____ Date of Birth _____

Street Address _____

City _____ State _____ Zip _____

Home Phone _____ Work Phone _____

Cell Phone _____

Physician Name _____

Physician Address _____

Physician Phone Number _____

Health Insurance Carrier _____

Group and/or Policy Number _____

Employer _____

Employer Address _____

Employer Phone Number_____

Emergency Contact_____

Relationship_____

Phone Number _____

Alternate Emergency Contact _____

Relationship_____

Phone Number _____

Patient Treatment Information

I am currently experiencing the following symptoms (circle all that apply):

Extreme head pain   Nausea   Sensitivity to sound

Sensitivity to light   Other

On a scale of 1 (lowest) to 10 (highest), my head pain severity is:

_____

I have taken the following medications:

_____

Drug Name / Dose / When Taken

_____

Drug Name / Dose / When Taken

_____

Drug Name / Dose / When Taken

_____

Other

Other prescription medications I take (name and dosage)

_____

Other OTC medications, vitamins, or supplements I take (name and dosage)

_____

Allergies

_____

Other nonmigraine health conditions

_____

Patient Name _____

Patient Signature _____

Date _____

Physician Emergency Treatment Form

My patient_____is a diagnosed migraineur, or migraine sufferer. He/she uses the medications indicated below to provide abortive and/or preventive treatment for migraine. My patient sometimes experiences severe migraine attacks that do not respond to the prescribed care regimen and require emergency treatment.

Patient Information

Patient Name _____

Date of Birth_____Date of Diagnosis_____

Current medications used for migraine prevention (name and dosage): _____

_____

Current medications used for acute treatment of migraine pain:

Other pain medications:_____

_____

Drugs and therapies proven ineffective for my patient's

migraines: _____

Medication allergies:_____

For emergency treatment, I suggest the following:_____

_____

Physician Information

Physician Name_____

Signature _____

Office Address_____

Office Phone Number_____

Migraine Glossary

Abdominal migraine
Most common in children, abdominal migraine is characterized by bouts of abdominal pain, nausea, and vomiting that can last for up to seventy-two hours.

Abortive medications
Also called rescue therapy; second-line treatments used to treat migraine acutely when a standard drug regimen does not work and migraine pain is severe. May include narcotics or opioid analgesics.

Acupuncture
A Traditional Chinese Medicine (TCM) treatment involving the placement of thin, disposable needles just under the skin, targeted to locations on the body known as "acupoints." The goal of acupuncture is to harmonize the energy flow within the body.

Acute treatment
An analgesic, or pain-relieving, medication or therapy that is taken when a migraine begins. It is designed to stop or alleviate the pain and other symptoms of a migraine attack.

Amines
Substances derived from amino acids that include tyramine, histamine and beta-phenylethylamine that may act as migraine triggers. They are found in many food products.

Analgesics
Pain-relieving over-the-counter or prescription medications used in the acute treatment of migraine.

Aneurysm
A weakened blood vessel wall that may be distended and is in danger of rupture, causing hemorrhage, or bleeding on the brain. Severe headache is one symptom of an aneurysm.

Aura
A group of changes that proceed a migraine headache, including visual, sensory, and cognitive changes, and last anywhere from five minutes to one hour. The most common type of aura is visual. This often occurs as flickering spots (photopsia), zigzag lines (teichopsia, or fortification spectrum), or areas of loss of vision (scotoma).

Basilar artery migraine
A migraine with aura caused by dilation of the basilar artery, which supplies blood to the brainstem. It has a specific aura profile and the migraine pain affects both sides of the head.

Biofeedback
A system of monitoring your body's biological signals, such as temperature, heart rate, and muscle tension, and learning how to regulate those functions through relaxation and visualization techniques.

Cluster headache
Intense and often excruciating pain in and around one eye that is accompanied by one-sided facial symptoms such as flushing, congestion, and swollen eye. These headaches occur in distinct patterns of close and frequent attacks, or clusters, of two weeks to three months that are followed by headache-free "remission" periods that can last anywhere from a month to several years.

Cortical spreading depression (CSD)
Misfiring of the neurons in the cortex of the brain that is thought to trigger both migraine headache, and the frequently accompanying aura and visual symptoms.

Endorphins
Natural painkillers produced by the body in times of pain and exertion.

Estrogen
A female sex hormone. Continuous high levels of estrogen may be associated with a decreased occurrence of migraine, while low levels, or sudden fluctuations in estrogen levels, are associated with an increase in migraine activity.

Hemiplegic migraine
A severe but rare migraine with aura that causes weakness or paralysis on one side of the body and can result in coma.

Histamine
An amine that is a derivative of amino acid and is a potential trigger for migraine attacks. Histamines are present in some foods naturally, including eggplant, spinach, and certain species of fish. They are also found in foods and drinks that ferment, such as vinegars, wine and beer, and sauerkraut.

Menstrual migraine
Migraine that is directly related to the menstrual cycle with no other identifiable triggers.

Migraine with aura
Migraine with aura is sometimes referred to as a *classic migraine*. The most common type of aura is visual. Migraine with aura is experienced by roughly 20 percent of all migraineurs.

Migraine without aura
Migraine without aura is sometimes called common migraine. Around 80 percent of migraineurs have migraine without the "early warning system" of the aura. Some people with this type of migraine may experience a prodrome—a group of physical and/or emotional symptoms occurring up

to seventy-two hours before a migraine headache.

MSG (monosodium glutamate)
Most well-known as an additive in Chinese food, MSG is found in seasonings, sauces, Parmesan cheese, and meat tenderizers and is a migraine trigger for many people.

Neurologist
A physician who specializes in diseases and disorders of the central and peripheral nervous system—including the brain, spinal cord, nerves, and muscles.

Neurotransmitter
A brain chemical that helps facilitate the transfer of nerve impulses, or electrical signals, between neurons (nerve cells).

Nitrates
Drugs prescribed to patients with angina and congestive heart failure. They dilate, or open, the blood vessels, which can cause vascular headache and facial flushing in some people.

Nitrites
Sodium nitrite is used as a preservative in many processed meats, including hot dogs and lunchmeat. The additive triggers attacks in many migraineurs.

NSAIDs
Nonsteroidal anti-inflammatory drugs. NSAIDS are used in both acute and preventative migraine treatment.

Phenylethylamine
A vasoconstrictor found in chocolate that may trigger migraines for some people.

Placebo
A clinically inactive drug or therapy usually used to treat subjects in the control group of a controlled clinical trial to provide a baseline for the efficacy of another treatment.

Preventative medications
Also called prophylactics, these drugs help to prevent a migraine attack.

Primary headache disorder
Headaches that are not symptomatic of another medical condition but exist independently. Examples of primary headache disorders include migraine and cluster headaches.

Prodrome
A group of physical and/or emotional symptoms occurring up to seventy-two hours before a migraine headache.

Progesterone
A female sex hormone.

Postdrome
Also called a headache hangover. A constellation of symptoms that follow the active migraine attack and may include fatigue, cognitive difficulties, mood change, dizziness, weakness, and an ongoing low-grade headache. The postdrome may last anywhere from a few hours to more than a day.

Rebound headache
Also called medication overuse headache. Overuse of some acute migraine medications can result in more frequent, and sometimes more intense, headache episodes.

Retinal (or Ocular) migraine

A type of migraine caused by nerve cell stimulation at the back of the brain, which can result in blindness or blurred vision in one eye.

Secondary headache

Headaches that are symptomatic of another medical condition. Some secondary causes of chronic headaches include high blood pressure, infections, stroke, and meningitis

Serotonin (5-HT)

A neurotransmitter, or brain chemical, that helps to regulate mood, appetite, sleep, and other brain/body functions. Decreased levels of serotonin are associated with migraine.

Sinus headache

Persistent head pain under the eyes and at the cheekbone, sometimes extending down into the top half of the mouth. Sinus headache may be one sided or occur on both sides of the face. Allergies, infections, and the common cold can all cause swelling and pressure buildup in the sinus cavity, and this inflammation is called sinusitis. Sometimes, a structural problem within the sinus and/or nasal cavities can cause pressure and subsequent sinus headache.

Sleep hygiene

The practice of getting regular, healthy amounts of sleep. Sleep hygiene is an important preventative strategy in migraine treatment.

Status migrainosus

A severe migraine attack lasting more than seventy-two hours.

Tension-type headache (TTH)

The most common type of primary headache disorder. The pain of a tension-type headache is often described as a tight band encircling the top of the head, mild to moderate in severity. It differs from migraine and cluster headache in that it is felt on both sides of the head and there is no nausea involved. A TTH lasts from thirty minutes to seven days. While a TTH may infrequently cause hypersensitivity to light or sound, as a migraine does, only one of these symptoms usually occurs (not both together as happens frequently with migraine).

Transient ischemic attack (TIA)

Also known as "ministroke," a TIA occurs when blood flow to the brain is diminished. The warning signs of TIA are the same as those of stroke—weakness, numbness, confusion, vision loss, difficulty speaking, severe headache—except they disappear in anywhere from a few minutes to a few hours, with all symptoms resolved within twenty-four hours. Because all of these are also found in migraine, there is a possibility of misdiagnosing TIA as migraine or vice versa.

Trigeminal nerve

The fifth cranial nerve, the largest nerve of the head and the gatekeeper for the nerve conduction that supplies sensation to the face.

Trigger

Something that sets off a migraine attack. Triggers may be something you encounter in your environment, such as food and drink additives, odors, or cigarettes, or a biological change in your body, such as changing levels of hormones. Triggers are very individual, and what prompts a migraine attack in one person may not have any impact on another. Identifying and avoiding triggers is a major component of migraine prevention.

Tyramine

An amino acid formed by the breakdown of proteins that is also a migraine trigger. Many foods that are aged, such as hard cheeses and fermented or pickled foods, contain tyramine, as do smoked meats, chocolate, soy sauce, onions, and nuts.

Vasoconstriction

A narrowing or constricting of a blood vessel.

Vasodilatation

A swelling or widening of a blood vessel.

INDEX

The Everything Health Guide to Migraines

Psychological triggers, 225
Puberty, 151–52

Race, 10
Raynaud's disease, 274–75
Rebound headaches, 98–99
Recovery. *See* Postdrome
Relaxation, 103–4, 117, 170, 191,
    226–27. *See also* Biofeedback
RELIEF mnemonic, 47–48
Retinal migraine, 7

School, triggers and
    treatment at, 173–75
Seasonal triggers, 81
Sensory triggers, 84–85, 165–66
Sexual activity, 193–95
Silent migraines, 178–79
Sinus/nasal problems, 25–26
Sleep, 20, 74–75, 99–100, 276
    children and, 138, 169–70, 176
    prevention and, 139, 189–91, 224
    recovery and, 137–39
Smoking, 20, 37, 74, 86,
    152, 156, 186
Social Security disability, 249–50
Socioeconomic status, 10, 12
Stress
    in children, 164, 167
    management of, 222–23
    during recovery, 139–40
    as trigger, 14, 75–76, 102
Stroke, 13, 29–30, 266–69
Sumatriptan, 21
Surgery, cluster headaches
    and, 22–23
Sweeteners, as triggers, 238–40

Temporal arteritis, 32
Tension headaches, 23–25
Transcranial magnetic
    stimulation (TMS), 281–83
Transient ischemic attack
    (TIA). *See* Stroke

Travel tips, 82–83, 142–43, 200–202
Treatment
    of cluster headaches, 21–23, 181
    of tension headaches, 25
Treatment, of migraines
    alternative and complementary
        medicine, 119–33
    antinausea medicines, 96–98
    to avoid rebound
        headaches, 98–99
    in children, 167–73
    future of, 279–92
    in men, 186–87
    for pain relief, 89–104
    prophylactic, 105–17
    in women, 154–55
Trexima, 280
Trigeminal autonomic
    cephalgias (TACs), 18
Triptans, 8, 94–96, 112,
    154–55, 168, 172, 181

Urine tests, 42

Valporic acid, 181
Verapamil, 22
Vitamin B2 (riboflavin), 119–21
Volproic acid, 22

Weather triggers, 79–80, 198–200
Women, 147–60
Work issues, 140, 142,
    195–98, 247–53

Yoga, 226–27

Zolmatriptan, 21